The Gut Switch

The Harmony Within: Nurturing Your Gut for Optimal Health

By Umesh M Pherwani

Dedication

To my Dad with everlasting love and heartfelt gratitude

Prologue

The Harmony Within: Nurturing Your Gut for Optimal Health

In the fast-paced world we inhabit, with its constant demands and ever-evolving challenges, maintaining our health and well-being has become more crucial than ever. While we often focus on external factors like exercise and skincare, we tend to overlook an essential aspect of our overall health—our gut. Hidden within us lies a bustling metropolis, teeming with trillions of microorganisms, collectively known as the gut microbiome. This intricate ecosystem plays a fundamental role in our well-being, influencing not only our digestive health but also our mental and immune functions.

Welcome to 'The Gut Switch' - Harmony Within: Nurturing Your Gut for Optimal Health." In this book, we embark on a journey to explore the wonders of our gut and understand the profound impact it has on our lives. We will delve into the intricate relationship between our gut and various aspects of our physical and mental well-being. By the end of this journey, you will have a deeper appreciation for your gut's vital role and gain practical knowledge to nurture it for optimal health.

Chapter by chapter, we will navigate the complex world of gut health, unraveling its mysteries and equipping you with valuable insights. We begin with Chapter 1, "Understanding Your Gut," where we lay the foundation by delving into the fascinating world of the gut microbiome. We explore the symbiotic relationship between the bacteria residing within us and the various roles they play in maintaining our health. Additionally, we uncover the remarkable connection between our gut and brain, highlighting the gut-brain axis and its influence on our mental well-being.

In Chapter 2, "Nurturing Your Gut with Nutrition," we shift our focus to the importance of a gut-friendly diet. We delve into the power of probiotics, beneficial bacteria that can bolster our gut health. You will discover how prebiotics, found in certain foods, serve as nourishment for these friendly microbes. Furthermore, we explore the wonders of fermented foods and their potential to promote a thriving gut environment. Lastly, we dive into the delicate balance of macro and micronutrients necessary for optimal gut health. Healing our gut takes center stage in Chapter 3, aptly titled "Healing Your Gut." We shed light on gut inflammation, a common issue that can disrupt the delicate balance within our digestive system. Understanding the causes and consequences of leaky gut syndrome, we then explore strategies to restore gut integrity and repair the gut lining. Additionally, we delve into gut-healing diets and the potential benefits of herbs and supplements in nurturing our gut.

The connection between the gut and mind takes the spotlight in Chapter 4, "The Gut-Mind Connection." We explore the profound influence of gut health on mental well-being, including the impact of stress, anxiety, and sleep disturbances. We unravel the concept of mindful eating and its role in nourishing both the gut and the mind. By the end of this chapter, you will gain insights into how emotional balance intertwines with gut health.

Chapter 5, "Lifestyle Factors for a Healthy Gut," sheds light on the lifestyle choices that can support gut health. We examine the relationship between exercise and gut harmony, exploring how physical activity contributes to a thriving digestive system. Additionally, we discuss the importance of sleep and circadian rhythms in maintaining a balanced gut environment. Stress management techniques and the influence of environmental factors on gut health are also explored. Lastly, we uncover the transformative power of mind-body practices in fostering gut well-being.

In Chapter 6, "Gut Health and Digestive Disorders," we turn our attention to the common gastrointestinal conditions that can hinder our gut health. We shed light on Irritable Bowel Syndrome (IBS), Inflammatory Bowel

In chapter 7 we go into Gut health across the lifespan. In chapter 8 we dive into gut health and weight management. In chapter 9 we explore gut health and immunity. Chapter 10 exposes the effects of sugar on our gut health.chapter 11 explores the effects of gluten on gut health and the co relation between gut health and depression.

Table of Contents:

Introduction

Chapter 1

<u>Understanding Your Gut</u>

1.1 The Marvelous Microbiome

Deep within the intricate folds of our digestive system lies an astonishing universe, teeming with trillions of microorganisms that make up our gut microbiome. The gut microbiome, an ecosystem of bacteria, viruses, fungi, and other microbes, is a fascinating and essential component of our overall health and well-being. In this chapter, "Understanding Your Gut," we embark on a journey to unravel the mysteries of the gut microbiome, exploring its composition, functions, and the profound influence it holds over our lives.

The Microbial Metropolis:

Within our gut, a bustling metropolis of microorganisms thrives, constituting a diverse and dynamic community. These microscopic inhabitants, collectively known as the gut microbiota, form a complex ecosystem that interacts with our bodies in countless ways. Comprised of hundreds of different species, the gut microbiota contributes to vital functions such as digestion, nutrient absorption, immune system regulation, and even the synthesis of certain vitamins.

The Birth of a Microbiome:

From the moment we take our first breath, our gut microbiome begins to develop and shape our health. While the womb was once believed to be a sterile environment, recent research has revealed that microbes can be transferred from mother to child before and during birth. This early colonization sets the stage for the establishment of a diverse and balanced gut microbiome.

Factors Influencing Gut Microbiome Composition:

The composition of our gut microbiome is influenced by various factors, including genetics, diet, environment, and early life experiences. Genetic predispositions may affect the types of bacteria that thrive in our gut, while dietary choices and nutrient availability provide the necessary resources for specific microbial populations to flourish. Additionally, environmental factors such as exposure to antibiotics, pollutants, and stress can impact the delicate balance of our gut microbiota.

Functions of the Gut Microbiome:

Beyond its role in digestion, the gut microbiome performs a myriad of essential functions. One of its primary tasks is to break down complex carbohydrates that our bodies cannot digest on their own, producing beneficial byproducts such as short-chain fatty acids that nourish the cells lining our intestinal walls. Furthermore, the gut microbiome plays a crucial role in training and modulating our immune system, ensuring its responsiveness while preventing overreactions.

The Gut-Brain Axis:

The gut microbiome is intricately connected to our brain through a bidirectional communication network known as the gut-brain axis. This pathway allows for constant information exchange between the gut and the central nervous system. The gut microbiota produces various molecules, including neurotransmitters and metabolites, that can influence brain function and behavior. Conversely, our emotions, stress levels, and dietary choices can shape the composition and activity of our gut microbiota.

Intuition and the Gut:

Beyond its physiological functions, the gut has long been associated with intuition and instinctive feelings. Phrases such as "gut feeling" and "butterflies in the stomach" reflect the connection between our gut and our intuitive senses. Emerging research suggests that this connection may be attributed to the extensive network of nerves embedded in our gut walls, known as the enteric nervous system. This "second brain" within our gut can independently regulate certain digestive processes and communicate with our primary brain.

As we conclude this exploration into the marvelous world of the gut microbiome, we begin to grasp the intricacy and importance of this hidden ecosystem. Our gut is far more than a mere organ responsible for digestion; it is a living community that profoundly influences our physical and mental well-being. Understanding the composition, functions, and connections of the gut microbiome lays the foundation for nurturing a healthy gut and unlocking the vast potential it holds for our overall health.

1.2: Gut-Brain Axis: Exploring the Connection

The gut-brain axis, a complex and bidirectional communication network between our gut and brain, serves as a vital link connecting our digestive system with our mental and emotional well-being. In this chapter, "Gut-Brain Axis: Exploring the Connection," we delve into the fascinating interplay between our gut and brain, uncovering the mechanisms behind this intricate relationship and understanding how it influences our emotions, cognition, and overall mental health.

The Communication Pathways:

The gut-brain axis operates through multiple communication pathways, allowing constant information exchange between the gut and the brain. One key channel is the vagus nerve, a major nerve that connects the brainstem to various organs, including the digestive system. This nerve facilitates bidirectional communication, enabling signals to travel back and forth between the gut and brain. Additionally, chemical messengers, such as hormones, neurotransmitters, and microbial metabolites, play a crucial role in relaying information and modulating the gut-brain axis.

The Enteric Nervous System (ENS):

Within the walls of our gut resides a vast network of nerves known as the enteric nervous system (ENS). Often referred to as the "second brain," the ENS operates independently of the central nervous system and plays a vital role in regulating gut functions. This intricate network of neurons controls digestion, nutrient absorption, and gastrointestinal motility, and it can communicate with the brain via the vagus nerve, shaping our overall gut-brain connection.

Neurotransmitters and the Gut:

Neurotransmitters, chemical messengers that facilitate communication between neurons, are not limited to the brain alone. In fact, an estimated 90% of serotonin, a key neurotransmitter associated with mood regulation, is produced in the gut. This finding highlights the significance of the gut in influencing our emotional state. Other neurotransmitters, such as gamma-aminobutyric acid (GABA) and dopamine, also play a role in the gut-brain axis, contributing to the regulation of stress, anxiety, and reward responses.

Microbiota-Gut-Brain Communication:

The gut microbiota, the collection of microorganisms residing in our gut, has emerged as a crucial player in the gut-brain axis. These microbes produce an array of compounds that can influence brain function and behavior. For instance, certain strains of bacteria produce neurotransmitters, such as gamma-aminobutyric acid (GABA) and serotonin, which can modulate mood and anxiety levels. Furthermore, microbial metabolites, such as short-chain fatty acids, have been shown to impact brain health and cognition.

Influence on Mental Health:

The gut-brain axis has a profound impact on our mental health and the development of psychiatric disorders. Research suggests that disruptions in the gut microbiota composition, known as dysbiosis, may be linked to conditions such as depression, anxiety, and even neurodevelopmental disorders like autism spectrum disorder. Understanding and nurturing a healthy gut microbiome may hold promise for managing and preventing mental health conditions.

Stress, Emotions, and the Gut:

Stress and emotions can significantly impact the gut-brain axis. The gut is equipped with receptors for stress hormones, and exposure to chronic or acute stress can disrupt gut function, alter the composition of the gut microbiota, and impair the integrity of the intestinal barrier. Conversely, a healthy gut microbiota can help regulate the body's stress response and mitigate the impact of stress on mental health.

Modulating the Gut-Brain Axis:

Various lifestyle and dietary factors can influence the gut-brain axis and promote a healthy connection between the gut and brain. Strategies such as regular exercise, stress management techniques, and mind-body practices like meditation and yoga have been

1.3: Gut Health and Overall Well-being

The health of our gut has far-reaching implications for our overall well-being. In this chapter, "Gut Health and Overall Well-being," we explore the intricate connections between gut health and various aspects of our physical, mental, and emotional well-being. Understanding the profound impact of gut health on overall wellness empowers us to make informed choices and take proactive steps to nurture and maintain a healthy gut.

Digestive Health:

A healthy gut is the foundation of good digestive health. The gut plays a crucial role in breaking down food, absorbing nutrients, and eliminating waste. When the gut microbiome is in balance, digestion is efficient, and nutrient absorption is optimized. However, imbalances in the gut microbiota can lead to digestive issues such as bloating, gas, constipation, or diarrhea. Nurturing a healthy gut microbiome is essential for maintaining optimal digestive function.

Immune Function:

The gut is intricately linked to our immune system, serving as a primary line of defense against pathogens. Approximately 70% to 80% of our immune cells reside in the gut-associated lymphoid tissue (GALT). The gut microbiota plays a vital role in training and regulating our immune system, helping to distinguish between harmless substances and potential threats. A healthy gut supports a robust immune response, helping to defend against infections, allergies, and autoimmune disorders.

Inflammation and Chronic Diseases:

Chronic inflammation is at the root of many chronic diseases, including cardiovascular disease, diabetes, obesity, and certain types of cancer. The gut microbiota plays a significant role in modulating inflammation throughout the body. Imbalances in the gut microbiome can lead to increased gut permeability, allowing harmful substances to enter the bloodstream and trigger systemic inflammation. Nurturing a healthy gut through diet, lifestyle, and targeted interventions can help reduce inflammation and lower the risk of chronic diseases.

Mental Health and Mood:

The gut-brain axis, the communication pathway between the gut and the brain, has a profound impact on mental health and mood regulation. Research has shown that imbalances in the gut microbiota are associated with an increased risk of mental health disorders such as depression, anxiety, and stress-related conditions. Serotonin, a neurotransmitter involved in mood regulation, is primarily produced in the gut. A healthy gut microbiome is crucial for maintaining optimal brain function and promoting positive mental well-being.

Sleep Quality:

Sleep is essential for overall well-being, and the gut can influence sleep quality in various ways. The gut microbiota produces molecules that can influence sleep patterns and circadian rhythms. Disruptions in the gut microbiome have been linked to sleep disturbances, such as insomnia and sleep apnea. Additionally, conditions such as

gastroesophageal reflux disease (GERD) and irritable bowel syndrome (IBS) can interfere with sleep quality. By nurturing a healthy gut, we can support restful sleep and improve overall sleep hygiene.
Skin Health:
The gut-skin axis highlights the relationship between gut health and the condition of our skin. The gut microbiota plays a role in modulating inflammation and immune responses that can impact skin health. Imbalances in the gut microbiome have been associated with skin conditions such as acne, eczema, and psoriasis. By addressing gut health, we can potentially improve skin conditions and promote a healthy complexion.
Energy Levels and Vitality:
The state of our gut has a direct impact on our energy levels and vitality. When the gut microbiota is in balance, it aids in the efficient breakdown and absorption of nutrients, providing the necessary energy for optimal functioning. However, imbalances in the gut can lead to nutrient deficiencies and decreased energy production. By prioritizing gut health through a nourishing diet and lifestyle,

1.4: Unveiling the Gut's Role in Immunity

The gut, often referred to as the "second brain," is not only responsible for digestion but also plays a crucial role in our immune system. In this chapter, "Unveiling the Gut's Role in Immunity," we delve into the intricate connections between the gut and our immune system. We explore how the gut microbiota, gut-associated lymphoid tissue (GALT), and gut-immune interactions contribute to maintaining a strong and balanced immune response, protecting us against pathogens and promoting overall health.
The Gut Microbiota and Immune System:
The gut microbiota, a vast community of microorganisms residing in our intestines, has a profound impact on our immune system. These beneficial bacteria train and regulate

our immune response, helping to distinguish between harmful pathogens and harmless substances. The gut microbiota stimulates the production of antibodies, activates immune cells, and influences the development of immune tolerance. Imbalances in the gut microbiota can lead to dysregulation of the immune system, increasing the risk of allergies, autoimmune disorders, and infections.

Gut-Associated Lymphoid Tissue (GALT):

The gut-associated lymphoid tissue (GALT) is a network of immune cells, lymphoid follicles, and specialized tissues located in the gut. GALT acts as a surveillance system, detecting and responding to pathogens in the gut. It includes structures such as Peyer's patches, which house immune cells and facilitate antigen sampling. GALT plays a crucial role in educating and coordinating immune responses in the gut, ensuring an effective defense against pathogens while maintaining immune tolerance to harmless substances.

Intestinal Barrier Function:

The gut's immune system works in close collaboration with the intestinal barrier, a selectively permeable layer that separates the gut lumen from the rest of the body. The intestinal barrier prevents harmful substances, such as toxins and pathogens, from entering the bloodstream while allowing the absorption of essential nutrients. Specialized cells in the gut lining, such as enterocytes and goblet cells, contribute to the integrity and function of the intestinal barrier. Disruptions in the gut microbiota or intestinal barrier can compromise immune responses and lead to increased susceptibility to infections and inflammation.

Toll-like Receptors and Pattern Recognition Receptors:

Toll-like receptors (TLRs) and pattern recognition receptors (PRRs) are essential components of the gut's immune system. These receptors recognize specific patterns on pathogens, triggering immune responses to eliminate the invaders. TLRs are present on immune cells and intestinal epithelial cells, sensing the presence of bacteria, viruses, and other microorganisms. Activation of TLRs and PRRs leads to the production of cytokines and other immune mediators, initiating an immune response tailored to the specific pathogen encountered.

Mucosal Immunity:

Mucosal immunity refers to the immune responses that occur at mucosal surfaces, including the gut, respiratory tract, and genitourinary tract. The gut's mucosal immune system is uniquely designed to tolerate harmless substances, such as food antigens, while mounting strong defenses against pathogens. It relies on specialized immune cells, such as secretory IgA-producing plasma cells and T regulatory cells, to maintain immune balance and prevent excessive inflammation. A well-functioning mucosal immune system is crucial for protection against gut infections and maintaining overall immune health.

Probiotics and Immune Regulation:

Probiotics, beneficial bacteria that can be consumed through food or supplements, have gained attention for their potential immune-modulating effects. Certain strains of probiotics can enhance gut barrier function, promote the production of antimicrobial peptides, and regulate immune cell activity. Probiotics have been studied for their potential in preventing and managing conditions such as allergic diseases, inflammatory bowel diseases

1.5: Listening to Your Gut: Intuition and Gut Health

We often hear phrases like "trust your gut" or "listen to your intuition," suggesting that there is a deep connection between our gut and our inner wisdom. In this chapter, "Listening to Your Gut: Intuition and Gut Health," we explore the fascinating relationship between our gut health and our intuitive senses. We delve into the concept of gut intuition, the role of the enteric nervous system, and how nurturing our gut health can enhance our intuitive abilities and overall well-being.

The Enteric Nervous System (ENS) and Gut Intuition:

The enteric nervous system (ENS), often referred to as the "second brain," is a complex network of neurons that lines the walls of our gastrointestinal tract. This intricate system communicates with the central nervous system and plays a crucial role in regulating gut functions. Recent research has uncovered the ENS's involvement in intuitive processes and decision-making. The ENS has its own neural pathways and can send signals to the brain, influencing our emotions, instincts, and intuitive responses.

Gut Microbiota and Intuition:

The gut microbiota, the collection of microorganisms residing in our gut, also plays a significant role in our overall well-being, including our intuitive senses. Emerging evidence suggests that the gut microbiota can influence brain function and behavior, potentially affecting our intuition. The microbial metabolites produced by the gut microbiota, such as neurotransmitters and short-chain fatty acids, can modulate brain activity and cognition, potentially enhancing our intuitive abilities.

The Gut-Brain Axis and Intuitive Insights:

The gut-brain axis, the bidirectional communication system between our gut and brain, serves as a crucial link connecting our physical and mental health. The gut sends signals to the brain via neural pathways, hormones, and neurotransmitters, influencing our emotions, cognition, and intuitive processes. Imbalances in the gut microbiota or disruptions in the gut-brain axis can impact our intuitive insights, leading to a disconnect between our gut feelings and our conscious decision-making.

Intuition as a Guide to Gut Health:

Our intuitive senses can also serve as a guide to our gut health. The gut has a remarkable ability to communicate its needs and imbalances through intuitive signals. Intuitive sensations such as gut feelings, hunches, or visceral reactions can provide valuable insights into our overall well-being. By learning to listen to these intuitive signals and developing a deeper connection with our gut, we can identify potential dietary triggers, allergens, or stressors that may be impacting our gut health.

Emotional Intelligence and Gut Health:

Emotional intelligence, the ability to understand and manage our emotions, is closely tied to our gut health and intuitive abilities. The gut-brain axis plays a significant role in regulating our emotions and mood. By nurturing our gut health, we can promote emotional resilience, enhance self-awareness, and improve our ability to trust and act upon our intuitive insights. Developing emotional intelligence allows us to make choices that support our gut health and overall well-being.

Intuitive Eating and Gut Health:

Intuitive eating, a mindful and intuitive approach to nourishing our bodies, aligns perfectly with the concept of listening to our gut. By paying attention to our body's hunger and satiety cues, we can foster a healthy relationship with food and support our gut health. Intuitive eating encourages us to trust our internal cues rather than relying on external rules or restrictions. It allows us to make food choices that nourish our bodies and promote optimal gut function.

Cultivating Gut Intuition:

Cultivating gut intuition is a journey that involves nurturing our gut health and developing our self-awareness. It requires us to slow down, listen to our body's signals, and pay attention to the subtle messages from our gut. Practices such as mindfulness, meditation, journaling, and gut-directed exercises can help us deepen our connection with our gut and strengthen our intuitive senses. By fostering a harmonious relationship between our gut and intuition, we can tap into our inner wisdom and make choices that support our overall well-being.

Our gut health and intuition are intricately intertwined, forming a profound connection that influences our physical, mental, and emotional well-being. By understanding and nurturing our gut health, we can enhance our intuitive abilities, trust our gut feelings, and make choices that promote optimal health and vitality. Listening to our gut becomes not just a metaphorical concept but a practical approach to living a balanced and fulfilled life. In the next chapters, we will explore practical strategies and lifestyle changes to nurture our gut and enhance our overall well-being.

Chapter 2

Nurturing Your Gut with Nutrition

2.1 The Power of Probiotics

Nutrition plays a vital role in nurturing and maintaining a healthy gut. In this chapter, "The Power of Probiotics," we delve into the world of beneficial bacteria and explore how these probiotics can positively impact our gut health. We uncover the science behind probiotics, their mechanisms of action, and the potential benefits they offer for our digestive system and overall well-being.

Understanding Probiotics:

Probiotics are live microorganisms that, when consumed in adequate amounts, confer health benefits on the host. These beneficial bacteria can be found in various food sources or taken as supplements. The most common types of probiotics belong to the Lactobacillus and Bifidobacterium genera, but other strains, such as Saccharomyces boulardii, are also utilized. Probiotics work by colonizing the gut and interacting with the gut microbiota, promoting a healthy balance of bacteria.

Restoring Gut Microbial Balance:

Our gut microbiota is a complex ecosystem comprising trillions of microorganisms. When this delicate balance is disrupted by factors such as poor diet, stress, or antibiotic use, it can lead to dysbiosis—a state of microbial imbalance associated with various digestive issues. Probiotics can help restore this balance by displacing harmful bacteria, supporting the growth of beneficial bacteria, and enhancing the diversity of the gut microbiota.

Enhancing Digestive Function:

Probiotics play a crucial role in optimizing digestive function. They produce enzymes that aid in the breakdown of complex carbohydrates, proteins, and fats, facilitating better nutrient absorption. Probiotics also help regulate gut motility, promoting regular bowel movements and reducing the risk of constipation or diarrhea. By enhancing digestive function, probiotics contribute to overall gut health and improve gastrointestinal comfort.

Supporting Immune Function:

A significant portion of our immune system resides in the gut, making the gut microbiota a key player in immune function. Probiotics can stimulate the production of antimicrobial peptides, enhance the function of immune cells, and modulate the inflammatory response. By supporting a healthy gut microbiota, probiotics help strengthen our immune defenses, reducing the risk of infections and promoting overall immune health.

Alleviating Digestive Disorders:

Probiotics have shown promise in alleviating various digestive disorders. In conditions such as irritable bowel syndrome (IBS), inflammatory bowel disease (IBD), and antibiotic-associated diarrhea, probiotics have been found to reduce symptoms, improve gut function, and support the healing of intestinal tissues. Certain strains of probiotics, such as Lactobacillus rhamnosus GG, have been extensively studied for their efficacy in these conditions.

Promoting Mental Well-being:

The gut-brain axis connects our gut and our central nervous system, influencing our mental health and well-being. Probiotics have been investigated for their potential to positively impact mental health conditions such as depression, anxiety, and stress. By modulating the gut microbiota and the production of neurotransmitters, probiotics can exert a positive influence on brain function, promoting a healthy mood and emotional balance.

Choosing the Right Probiotics:

Not all probiotics are created equal, and selecting the right strains and formulations is crucial for optimal benefits. Different probiotic strains have specific mechanisms of action and target different areas of gut health. Factors to consider when choosing probiotics include the strain's scientific evidence, viability, appropriate dosage, and compatibility with individual health conditions. Consulting with a healthcare professional can help determine the most suitable probiotic for individual needs.

Incorporating Probiotics into Your Diet:

Probiotics can be incorporated into the diet through various food sources or supplements. Fermented foods, such as yogurt, kefir, sauerkraut, and kimchi, naturally contain live probiotics. These foods not only provide probiotics but also offer additional nutrients and health benefits. Probiotic supplements are another option, providing a concentrated dose of specific strains. It's important to choose high-quality products and follow recommended dosage guidelines.

Probiotics are a valuable tool for nurturing our gut health and promoting overall well-being. These beneficial bacteria support digestive function, enhance immune response, alleviate digestive disorders, and even influence our mental well-being. By understanding the power of probiotics and incorporating them into our diet, we can take proactive steps toward optimizing our gut health. In the next chapters, we will explore further nutritional strategies and lifestyle changes to nourish our gut and foster optimal health.

2.2 Prebiotics: Fueling a Healthy Gut

While probiotics have gained considerable attention for their role in gut health, another essential component of a healthy gut ecosystem is prebiotics. In this chapter, "Prebiotics: Fueling a Healthy Gut," we explore the fascinating world of prebiotic fibers and their impact on nurturing our gut microbiota. We delve into the science behind prebiotics, their health benefits, and practical ways to incorporate them into our diet for optimal gut health.

Understanding Prebiotics:

Prebiotics are a type of dietary fiber that our bodies cannot digest. Instead, they serve as fuel for the beneficial bacteria in our gut, promoting their growth and activity. Prebiotics selectively stimulate the growth and activity of specific strains of bacteria, particularly those belonging to the Bifidobacterium and Lactobacillus genera. By nourishing these beneficial bacteria, prebiotics contribute to a balanced and diverse gut microbiota.

Types of Prebiotics:

The two most common types of prebiotics are inulin and fructooligosaccharides (FOS). Inulin is found in various plant-based foods such as chicory root, Jerusalem artichoke, and onions. FOS, on the other hand, is naturally present in foods like bananas, garlic, and asparagus. Both inulin and FOS serve as substrates for the fermentation process carried out by beneficial gut bacteria, leading to the production of short-chain fatty acids (SCFAs), which provide numerous health benefits.

Health Benefits of Prebiotics:

- Gut Microbiota Modulation: Prebiotics selectively promote the growth of beneficial bacteria, helping to restore and maintain a healthy gut microbiota. By nourishing these bacteria, prebiotics contribute to a diverse microbial community, which is associated with improved gut health and overall well-being.
- Enhanced Nutrient Absorption: The fermentation of prebiotics by gut bacteria produces SCFAs, such as acetate, propionate, and butyrate. SCFAs have been shown to improve the absorption of nutrients, particularly minerals like calcium and magnesium. By enhancing nutrient absorption, prebiotics support overall nutritional status and bone health.
- Improved Digestive Function: Prebiotics promote regular bowel movements and alleviate symptoms of constipation. The fermentation of prebiotics produces bulkier stools and increases the water content of the intestine, facilitating smoother passage of waste through the digestive tract.
- Immune System Support: A healthy gut microbiota is essential for a robust immune system. Prebiotics contribute to a favorable gut environment,

enhancing the growth of beneficial bacteria that interact with the gut-associated lymphoid tissue (GALT) and stimulate immune responses. By supporting immune function, prebiotics can help reduce the risk of infections and promote overall immune health.

- Reduced Inflammation: SCFAs produced during the fermentation of prebiotics have anti-inflammatory properties. They help maintain a balanced inflammatory response in the gut, preventing excessive inflammation that can contribute to conditions like inflammatory bowel disease (IBD) or irritable bowel syndrome (IBS).

Incorporating Prebiotics into Your Diet:

Including prebiotic-rich foods in your diet is an effective way to fuel a healthy gut. Some excellent sources of prebiotics include:

- Chicory Root: This root vegetable is a concentrated source of inulin, making it an excellent addition to your diet. It can be brewed as a tea or added to coffee as a prebiotic-rich alternative to traditional sweeteners.
- Jerusalem Artichoke: This knobby vegetable is rich in inulin and can be enjoyed roasted, steamed, or pureed into soups and stews.
- Onions and Garlic: These aromatic staples contain both inulin and FOS. Incorporate them into your cooking as flavor enhancers to reap the prebiotic benefits.
- Bananas: Unripe bananas are a great source of resistant starch, a type of prebiotic fiber that resists digestion in the small intestine and reaches the colon to fuel beneficial bacteria.
- Whole Grains: Oats, barley, and whole wheat are rich in prebiotic fibers. Enjoy a hearty bowl of oatmeal, opt for whole grain bread, or experiment with different whole grains in your meals.
- Legumes: Beans, lentils, and chickpeas are not only excellent sources of plant-based protein but also provide prebiotic fibers. Include these versatile legumes in soups, salads, or as a side dish.

Prebiotics are the fuel that nourishes our gut microbiota, promoting a healthy and balanced ecosystem. By selectively stimulating the growth of beneficial bacteria, prebiotics contribute to improved gut health, enhanced nutrient absorption, and a strengthened immune system. Incorporating prebiotic-rich foods into our diet allows us to fuel a healthy gut and support overall well-being. In the next chapters, we will continue our exploration of nutrition's role in nurturing our gut and fostering optimal health.

2.3 Fermented Foods: A Feast for Your Gut

Fermented foods have been part of human diets for centuries, and their consumption has been associated with numerous health benefits, particularly for the gut. In this chapter, "Fermented Foods: A Feast for Your Gut," we explore the world of these culinary delights and their impact on nurturing a healthy gut microbiota. We delve into the science behind fermentation, the benefits of fermented foods, and practical ways to incorporate them into our diet for optimal gut health.

Understanding Fermentation:

Fermentation is a metabolic process where microorganisms, such as bacteria or yeast, break down carbohydrates into simpler compounds like organic acids or alcohol. This process not only enhances the flavor, texture, and shelf life of foods but also promotes the growth of beneficial bacteria. During fermentation, these bacteria produce enzymes and probiotics that contribute to improved gut health and overall well-being.

Benefits of Fermented Foods:

- Probiotic Powerhouse: Fermented foods are rich in live beneficial bacteria, also known as probiotics. These probiotics, such as lactobacilli and bifidobacteria, help colonize the gut and enhance its microbial diversity. Consuming fermented foods regularly can contribute to a healthier gut microbiota, supporting digestion, nutrient absorption, and immune function.

- Improved Digestive Health: The fermentation process breaks down complex carbohydrates, making them easier to digest. Fermented foods can help alleviate digestive issues such as bloating, gas, and indigestion. They can also enhance the production of digestive enzymes, promoting optimal nutrient absorption and gut motility.
- Enhanced Nutrient Bioavailability: Fermentation can increase the bioavailability of certain nutrients. For example, fermented dairy products like yogurt or kefir enhance the absorption of calcium, while fermented vegetables increase the availability of vitamins and minerals. This means that incorporating fermented foods into our diet can maximize the nutritional benefits we receive from other foods.
- Gut Microbiota Balance: Fermented foods help maintain a balanced and diverse gut microbiota. The beneficial bacteria in these foods, such as lactobacilli and bifidobacteria, can outcompete harmful bacteria, creating an environment that supports optimal gut health. A balanced gut microbiota is associated with improved digestion, reduced inflammation, and enhanced immune function.
- Immune System Support: A significant portion of our immune system resides in the gut, and a healthy gut microbiota plays a crucial role in supporting immune function. Fermented foods can strengthen our immune defenses by promoting a favorable gut environment, modulating the inflammatory response, and enhancing the production of antimicrobial substances.

Incorporating Fermented Foods into Your Diet:

Integrating fermented foods into your daily diet is an excellent way to support your gut health. Here are some popular fermented foods to consider:

- Yogurt: Made from the fermentation of milk by lactic acid bacteria, yogurt is a well-known probiotic-rich food. Look for yogurt with live and active cultures, and choose unsweetened or minimally sweetened varieties for maximum benefits.

- Kefir: This fermented dairy beverage is similar to yogurt but has a thinner consistency and a tangy flavor. It contains a diverse range of probiotics and is rich in nutrients like calcium, protein, and B vitamins.
- Sauerkraut: Fermented cabbage is a traditional fermented food that is packed with probiotics and beneficial enzymes. Look for unpasteurized sauerkraut to ensure the presence of live cultures.
- Kimchi: A Korean staple, kimchi is a spicy fermented vegetable dish that typically includes cabbage, radishes, and various seasonings. It is a flavorful source of probiotics, vitamins, and antioxidants.
- Kombucha: This fermented tea beverage is made by fermenting sweetened tea with a symbiotic culture of bacteria and yeast (SCOBY). Kombucha is known for its probiotic content and refreshing taste.
- Miso: A traditional Japanese condiment, miso is made from fermented soybeans and grains. It adds depth of flavor to soups, stews, and marinades while providing probiotics and beneficial enzymes.
- Tempeh: Originating from Indonesia, tempeh is a fermented soybean product that is high in protein, fiber, and various nutrients. It has a nutty flavor and a firm texture, making it a versatile ingredient in plant-based cooking.

Fermented foods are not only delicious but also offer numerous health benefits, particularly for our gut. Their probiotic content, improved nutrient bioavailability, and support for a balanced gut microbiota make them a valuable addition to our diet. By incorporating fermented foods like yogurt, sauerkraut, and kefir, we can nourish our gut, enhance digestion, support our immune system, and promote overall well-being. In the next chapters, we will continue our exploration of nutrition's role in nurturing our gut and fostering optimal health.

2.4 Gut-Friendly Superfoods

Superfoods have gained popularity for their exceptional nutrient density and health benefits. In this chapter, "Gut-Friendly Superfoods," we explore a selection of nutrient-rich foods that not only provide essential vitamins and minerals but also support a healthy gut. We will dive into the science behind these superfoods, their specific gut-nurturing properties, and practical ways to incorporate them into our diet for optimal gut health.

Understanding Gut-Friendly Superfoods:

Gut-friendly superfoods are nutrient-dense foods that offer a variety of beneficial compounds that positively impact our gut health. These foods are typically rich in fiber, antioxidants, vitamins, and minerals that support digestive function, promote a diverse gut microbiota, and contribute to overall well-being.

Powerful Gut-Friendly Superfoods:

- Berries: Berries, such as blueberries, strawberries, and raspberries, are packed with antioxidants and fiber. The antioxidants help reduce inflammation in the gut, while the fiber provides nourishment for beneficial gut bacteria. Enjoy berries as a snack, in smoothies, or as a topping for oatmeal or yogurt.
- Leafy Greens: Dark leafy greens like spinach, kale, and Swiss chard are excellent sources of fiber, vitamins, and minerals. They promote regular bowel movements, provide prebiotic fiber for gut bacteria, and support overall digestive health. Incorporate leafy greens into salads, stir-fries, or smoothies.
- Flaxseeds: These tiny seeds are rich in fiber and omega-3 fatty acids, which have anti-inflammatory properties. The fiber content helps promote regular bowel movements and supports gut health. Grind flaxseeds before consuming them to enhance nutrient

absorption. Add them to smoothies, yogurt, or sprinkle them on salads or oatmeal.

- Chia Seeds: Like flaxseeds, chia seeds are an excellent source of fiber, omega-3 fatty acids, and antioxidants. They absorb liquid and form a gel-like substance in the gut, promoting healthy digestion and regular bowel movements. Enjoy chia seeds in puddings, smoothies, or as an egg substitute in baking.
- Fermented Soy: Fermented soy products like tempeh and miso provide plant-based protein, probiotics, and enzymes that support gut health. They can help balance gut bacteria and improve digestion. Use tempeh in stir-fries or as a meat substitute, and incorporate miso into soups, dressings, or marinades.
- Ginger: Ginger has long been used for its digestive benefits. It helps soothe the digestive system, reduce inflammation, and alleviate symptoms of indigestion and nausea. Enjoy ginger in teas, stir-fries, or grated into dishes for a flavorful and gut-nurturing kick.
- Turmeric: This vibrant yellow spice contains curcumin, a compound with powerful anti-inflammatory properties. It can help reduce inflammation in the gut and support digestive health. Add turmeric to curries, smoothies, or golden milk for a dose of gut-friendly goodness.
- Garlic: Garlic is known for its antimicrobial and immune-boosting properties. It can help promote a healthy balance of gut bacteria and support a robust immune system. Include garlic in your cooking, either raw or cooked, to add flavor and gut health benefits to your meals.
- Almonds: Almonds are packed with fiber, healthy fats, and vitamin E. They provide nourishment for beneficial gut bacteria and support overall gut health. Enjoy almonds as a snack, sprinkle them on salads, or use almond butter as a spread.
- Greek Yogurt: Greek yogurt is rich in protein and probiotics, making it a gut-friendly dairy option. The

probiotics in yogurt help promote a healthy gut microbiota and support digestion. Choose unsweetened or minimally sweetened varieties and add your favorite fruits or nuts for added flavor.

Incorporating Gut-Friendly Superfoods into Your Diet:

Now that we understand the gut-nurturing properties of these superfoods, let's explore some practical ways to incorporate them into our daily diet:

- Start your day with a gut-friendly smoothie by combining berries, leafy greens, chia seeds, and a scoop of Greek yogurt.
- Top your salads with flaxseeds, sliced almonds, and a drizzle of olive oil and lemon juice for a gut-healthy boost.
- Prepare flavorful stir-fries with fermented soy like tempeh, along with an array of colorful vegetables and aromatic spices like ginger and garlic.
- Snack on a handful of mixed nuts, including almonds, for a fiber and nutrient-rich treat.
- Experiment with turmeric in your cooking, adding it to curries, soups, or roasted vegetables for a burst of flavor and gut-nurturing benefits.

Gut-friendly superfoods offer a delicious and nutritious way to support our gut health. By incorporating these nutrient-dense foods like berries, leafy greens, flaxseeds, and fermented soy into our diet, we can promote digestive health, nourish our gut microbiota, and enhance overall well-being. The power of these foods lies not only in their individual benefits but also in their collective impact on our gut ecosystem. In the next chapters, we will continue exploring nutrition's role in nurturing our gut and fostering optimal health.

2.5 Finding Balance: Macro and Micronutrients for Gut Health

Achieving optimal gut health goes beyond incorporating specific foods into our diet. It also requires understanding the importance of balancing macro and micronutrients. In this chapter, "Finding Balance: Macro and Micronutrients for Gut Health," we explore the essential role that both macro and micronutrients play in supporting a healthy gut. We delve into the science behind these nutrients, their impact on gut health, and practical ways to ensure we achieve a well-rounded and nourishing diet for optimal gut health.

Understanding Macro and Micronutrients:

Macro and micronutrients are vital components of a healthy diet. Macro-nutrients include carbohydrates, proteins, and fats, which provide energy and support various bodily functions. Micronutrients, on the other hand, encompass vitamins and minerals, which are essential for numerous physiological processes.

The Gut-Macro and Micronutrient Connection:

- Carbohydrates: Carbohydrates are the primary energy source for our body and play a crucial role in gut health. Complex carbohydrates, found in whole grains, legumes, and vegetables, provide dietary fiber that feeds beneficial gut bacteria and supports regular bowel movements. Consuming a balanced amount of carbohydrates is essential for maintaining a healthy gut ecosystem.
- Proteins: Proteins are the building blocks of life and are necessary for the growth, repair, and maintenance of body tissues. They also play a role in maintaining a healthy gut lining. High-quality proteins, such as lean meats, poultry, fish, eggs, and plant-based sources like legumes and tofu, provide essential amino acids that support gut tissue integrity and immune function.
- Fats: Healthy fats are essential for the absorption of fat-soluble vitamins and the production of hormones. Omega-3 fatty acids, found in fatty fish, flaxseeds, and

walnuts, have anti-inflammatory properties that can benefit gut health. Incorporating sources of healthy fats, such as avocados, nuts, and olive oil, into our diet is crucial for a well-rounded approach to gut health.

- Vitamins: Vitamins are essential for various physiological functions, including gut health. Vitamin A supports the integrity of the gut lining, while vitamin D modulates the immune response in the gut. B vitamins, including folate and B12, are necessary for maintaining a healthy gut microbiota. Consuming a diverse range of fruits, vegetables, whole grains, and animal products can help ensure an adequate intake of essential vitamins.
- Minerals: Minerals are vital for enzymatic reactions, nerve function, and overall health. Zinc and magnesium, for example, are involved in maintaining the integrity of the gut lining and supporting immune function. Iron is necessary for the production of red blood cells, which transport oxygen to the gut and other tissues. Incorporating mineral-rich foods like leafy greens, nuts, seeds, and lean meats into our diet is essential for meeting our mineral needs.

Finding Balance in Your Diet:

Achieving a well-rounded and balanced diet is crucial for optimal gut health. Here are some practical tips to help you find the right balance of macro and micronutrients:

- Prioritize Whole Foods: Focus on consuming whole, unprocessed foods as the foundation of your diet. These foods provide a wide range of macro and micronutrients necessary for gut health.
- Include a Variety of Foods: Incorporate a diverse range of fruits, vegetables, whole grains, lean proteins, and healthy fats into your meals. This will ensure that you receive a broad spectrum of macro and micronutrients.
- Embrace Fiber-Rich Foods: Aim to include a good amount of fiber-rich foods like whole grains, legumes, fruits, and vegetables in your diet. Fiber supports healthy

digestion, feeds beneficial gut bacteria, and promotes regular bowel movements.
- Consider Portion Sizes: Pay attention to portion sizes to ensure you're consuming an appropriate amount of macro and micronutrients. Strive for balance and moderation in your meals.
- Consult with a Registered Dietitian: If you have specific dietary concerns or health conditions, consider consulting with a registered dietitian who can provide personalized guidance to help you achieve a balanced diet for optimal gut health.

Balancing macro and micronutrients is key to nourishing our gut and supporting optimal health. By understanding the role of carbohydrates, proteins, fats, vitamins, and minerals in gut health, we can make informed choices that benefit our overall well-being. Incorporate a variety of whole foods, prioritize fiber-rich options, and ensure proper portion sizes to achieve a balanced diet that supports gut health. In the next chapters, we will continue exploring nutrition's role in nurturing our gut and fostering optimal health.

 have been part of human diets for centuries, and their consumption has been associated with numerous health benefits, particularly for the gut. In this chapter, "Fermented Foods: A Feast for Your Gut," we explore the world of these culinary delights and their impact on nurturing a healthy gut microbiota. We delve into the science behind fermentation, the benefits of fermented foods, and practical ways to incorporate them into our diet for optimal gut health.

Understanding Fermentation:

Fermentation is a metabolic process where microorganisms, such as bacteria or yeast, break down carbohydrates into simpler compounds like organic acids or alcohol. This process not only enhances the flavor, texture, and shelf life of foods but also promotes the growth of beneficial bacteria. During fermentation, these bacteria produce enzymes and probiotics that contribute to improved gut health and overall well-being.

Benefits of Fermented Foods:

- Probiotic Powerhouse: Fermented foods are rich in live beneficial bacteria, also known as probiotics. These probiotics, such as lactobacilli and bifidobacteria, help colonize the gut and enhance its microbial diversity. Consuming fermented foods regularly can contribute to a healthier gut microbiota, supporting digestion, nutrient absorption, and immune function.
- Improved Digestive Health: The fermentation process breaks down complex carbohydrates, making them easier to digest. Fermented foods can help alleviate digestive issues such as bloating, gas, and indigestion. They can also enhance the production of digestive enzymes, promoting optimal nutrient absorption and gut motility.
- Enhanced Nutrient Bioavailability: Fermentation can increase the bioavailability of certain nutrients. For example, fermented dairy products like yogurt or kefir enhance the absorption of calcium, while fermented vegetables increase the availability of vitamins and minerals. This means that incorporating fermented foods into our diet can maximize the nutritional benefits we receive from other foods.
- Gut Microbiota Balance: Fermented foods help maintain a balanced and diverse gut microbiota. The beneficial bacteria in these foods, such as lactobacilli and bifidobacteria, can outcompete harmful bacteria, creating an environment that supports optimal gut health. A balanced gut microbiota is associated with improved digestion, reduced inflammation, and enhanced immune function.
- Immune System Support: A significant portion of our immune system resides in the gut, and a healthy gut microbiota plays a crucial role in supporting immune function. Fermented foods can strengthen our immune defenses by promoting a favorable gut environment, modulating the inflammatory response, and enhancing the production of antimicrobial substances.

Incorporating Fermented Foods into Your Diet:
Integrating fermented foods into your daily diet is an excellent way to support your gut health. Here are some popular fermented foods to consider:

- Yogurt: Made from the fermentation of milk by lactic acid bacteria, yogurt is a well-known probiotic-rich food. Look for yogurt with live and active cultures, and choose unsweetened or minimally sweetened varieties for maximum benefits.
- Kefir: This fermented dairy beverage is similar to yogurt but has a thinner consistency and a tangy flavor. It contains a diverse range of probiotics and is rich in nutrients like calcium, protein, and B vitamins.
- Sauerkraut: Fermented cabbage is a traditional fermented food that is packed with probiotics and beneficial enzymes. Look for unpasteurized sauerkraut to ensure the presence of live cultures.
- Kimchi: A Korean staple, kimchi is a spicy fermented vegetable dish that typically includes cabbage, radishes, and various seasonings. It is a flavorful source of probiotics, vitamins, and antioxidants.
- Kombucha: This fermented tea beverage is made by fermenting sweetened tea with a symbiotic culture of bacteria and yeast (SCOBY). Kombucha is known for its probiotic content and refreshing taste.
- Miso: A traditional Japanese condiment, miso is made from fermented soybeans and grains. It adds depth of flavor to soups, stews, and marinades while providing probiotics and beneficial enzymes.
- Tempeh: Originating from Indonesia, tempeh is a fermented soybean product that is high in protein, fiber, and various nutrients. It has a nutty flavor and a firm texture, making it a versatile ingredient in plant-based cooking.

Fermented foods are not only delicious but also offer numerous health benefits, particularly for our gut. Their probiotic content, improved nutrient bioavailability, and support for a balanced gut microbiota make them a valuable addition to our diet. By incorporating fermented foods like yogurt, sauerkraut, and kefir, we can nourish our gut, enhance digestion, support our immune system, and promote overall well-being. In the next chapters, we will continue our exploration of nutrition's role in nurturing our gut and fostering optimal health.

Chapter 3:

Healing Your Gut

3.1 Recognizing and Addressing Gut Inflammation

Gut inflammation can be a significant underlying factor in various gut-related disorders and can significantly impact overall health and well-being. In this chapter, "Recognizing and Addressing Gut Inflammation," we explore the causes, symptoms, and consequences of gut inflammation. We also discuss strategies and lifestyle modifications that can help reduce inflammation and promote gut healing for optimal health.

Understanding Gut Inflammation:

Inflammation is the body's natural response to injury or infection, aimed at protecting and repairing tissues. However, when inflammation becomes chronic or excessive, it can lead to detrimental effects on the gut and overall health. Gut inflammation can be triggered by various factors, including diet, stress, environmental toxins, food intolerances, and imbalances in the gut microbiota.

Signs and Symptoms of Gut Inflammation:

- Digestive Issues: Gut inflammation often manifests as digestive symptoms such as bloating, gas, abdominal pain, diarrhea, or constipation. These symptoms may be chronic or recurring.
- Food Sensitivities: Inflammation in the gut can lead to increased intestinal permeability, also known as "leaky gut." This can result in the development of food sensitivities or allergies, as undigested food particles and toxins leak into the bloodstream.
- Fatigue and Low Energy: Chronic gut inflammation can contribute to systemic inflammation, leading to fatigue, low energy levels, and a general feeling of malaise.

- Skin Problems: Inflammation in the gut can manifest on the skin, leading to conditions such as acne, eczema, or psoriasis.
- Joint Pain and Inflammation: Gut inflammation can trigger an immune response that affects joints, leading to joint pain, stiffness, and inflammation.

Addressing Gut Inflammation:

- Diet Modifications: Adopting an anti-inflammatory diet can be beneficial in reducing gut inflammation. Focus on consuming whole, unprocessed foods rich in antioxidants, healthy fats, and fiber. Minimize or eliminate processed foods, refined sugars, excessive alcohol, and potential trigger foods.
- Probiotics and Fermented Foods: Probiotics help restore the balance of beneficial gut bacteria, supporting gut health and reducing inflammation. Incorporate probiotic-rich foods like yogurt, kefir, sauerkraut, and kimchi into your diet.
- Managing Stress: Chronic stress can contribute to gut inflammation. Implement stress-management techniques such as meditation, deep breathing exercises, yoga, or engaging in hobbies to reduce stress levels.
- Sleep and Rest: Prioritize adequate sleep and rest to support overall healing and reduce inflammation.
- Identifying Food Triggers: Keep a food diary to identify potential trigger foods that may be causing or exacerbating gut inflammation. Consider working with a healthcare professional or registered dietitian to perform elimination diets or food sensitivity testing.
- Supporting Gut Repair: Include foods that support gut healing and repair, such as bone broth, aloe vera, slippery elm, and glutamine.
- Addressing Underlying Conditions: If gut inflammation persists or worsens, it is essential to seek medical attention to identify and address any underlying conditions that may be contributing to the inflammation.

Recognizing and addressing gut inflammation is crucial for promoting gut healing and overall health. By understanding the causes and symptoms of gut inflammation and implementing appropriate lifestyle modifications, dietary changes, and stress management techniques, we can reduce inflammation, restore gut health, and alleviate related symptoms. Healing the gut requires a holistic approach that encompasses nutrition, lifestyle choices, and targeted interventions. In the next chapters, we will continue our exploration of healing the gut and nurturing our overall well-being.

3.2 Leaky Gut Syndrome: Causes and Solutions

Leaky gut syndrome, also known as increased intestinal permeability, is a condition that has gained significant attention in recent years. It is characterized by a compromised intestinal barrier, allowing substances such as toxins, undigested food particles, and bacteria to leak from the gut into the bloodstream. In this chapter, "Leaky Gut Syndrome: Causes and Solutions," we explore the causes, symptoms, and consequences of leaky gut syndrome. We also discuss strategies and interventions that can help address this condition and promote gut healing for optimal health.

Understanding Leaky Gut Syndrome:

The intestinal lining serves as a barrier that selectively allows nutrients to be absorbed into the bloodstream while preventing harmful substances from entering. In the case of leaky gut syndrome, the tight junctions between the cells of the intestinal lining become compromised, allowing larger particles to pass through, triggering an immune response and inflammation.

Causes of Leaky Gut Syndrome:

- Poor Diet: Consuming a diet high in processed foods, refined sugars, unhealthy fats, and lacking in fiber and nutrient-dense foods can contribute to gut inflammation and compromise the integrity of the intestinal lining.

- Chronic Stress: Prolonged stress can impair gut function, disrupt the balance of gut bacteria, and contribute to increased intestinal permeability.
- Imbalance in Gut Microbiota: An imbalance in the gut microbiota, known as dysbiosis, can lead to gut inflammation and compromise the integrity of the intestinal barrier.
- Medications: Certain medications, such as nonsteroidal anti-inflammatory drugs (NSAIDs), antibiotics, and proton pump inhibitors (PPIs), can disrupt the gut microbiota and contribute to increased intestinal permeability.
- Environmental Factors: Exposure to environmental toxins, such as pesticides, pollutants, and heavy metals, can contribute to gut inflammation and compromise the integrity of the intestinal barrier.

Symptoms of Leaky Gut Syndrome:

- Digestive Issues: Leaky gut syndrome is often associated with digestive symptoms, including bloating, gas, abdominal pain, diarrhea, or constipation.
- Food Sensitivities: Increased intestinal permeability can lead to the development of food sensitivities or allergies, as larger particles leak into the bloodstream and trigger an immune response.
- Fatigue and Low Energy: Chronic inflammation resulting from leaky gut syndrome can lead to systemic inflammation, contributing to fatigue and low energy levels.
- Skin Conditions: Leaky gut syndrome has been linked to skin conditions such as acne, eczema, and psoriasis.
- Autoimmune Disorders: Some research suggests that leaky gut syndrome may be associated with the development or exacerbation of autoimmune disorders.

Addressing Leaky Gut Syndrome:

- Dietary Modifications: Adopting an anti-inflammatory diet that focuses on whole, unprocessed foods, rich in fiber, antioxidants, and healthy fats can help reduce inflammation and support gut healing.
- Gut-Healing Foods: Incorporate gut-healing foods such as bone broth, aloe vera, slippery elm, and glutamine into your diet to support the restoration of the intestinal lining.
- Probiotics and Fermented Foods: Probiotics help restore the balance of beneficial gut bacteria, supporting gut health and reducing inflammation. Include probiotic-rich foods like yogurt, kefir, sauerkraut, and kimchi in your diet.
- Stress Management: Implement stress-management techniques like meditation, deep breathing exercises, and regular physical activity to reduce stress levels and support gut healing.
- Gut Microbiota Support: Consider incorporating prebiotic-rich foods, such as onions, garlic, bananas, and asparagus, into your diet to nourish and promote the growth of beneficial gut bacteria.
- Identifying and Eliminating Triggers: Keep a food diary and work with a healthcare professional or registered dietitian to identify and eliminate potential trigger foods that may exacerbate leaky gut syndrome.
- Reduce Toxin Exposure: Minimize exposure to environmental toxins by choosing organic produce, using natural cleaning and personal care products, and avoiding unnecessary medications.

Leaky gut syndrome can have a significant impact on gut health and overall well-being. Understanding the causes, symptoms, and consequences of this condition empowers us to take proactive steps towards addressing it. By implementing dietary modifications, incorporating gut-healing foods, managing stress, supporting the gut microbiota, and reducing toxin exposure, we can promote gut healing and restore the integrity of the intestinal barrier.

Healing leaky gut syndrome requires a comprehensive approach that addresses the underlying causes and supports overall gut health. In the next chapters, we will continue our exploration of healing the gut and nurturing optimal health.

3.3 Restoring Gut Integrity: Repairing the Gut Lining

Restoring gut integrity is a crucial aspect of healing the gut and addressing conditions like leaky gut syndrome. The gut lining serves as a protective barrier, and when it becomes compromised, it can lead to various health issues. In this chapter, "Restoring Gut Integrity: Repairing the Gut Lining," we will explore strategies and interventions aimed at repairing and strengthening the gut lining. By focusing on targeted approaches, we can promote gut healing, reduce inflammation, and optimize overall gut health.

Understanding the Gut Lining:

The gut lining consists of a single layer of cells that form a barrier between the contents of the gut and the bloodstream. This barrier selectively allows nutrients to be absorbed while preventing harmful substances from entering. The cells are tightly connected through junctions that maintain the integrity of the gut lining. When these junctions become compromised, the gut lining becomes permeable, allowing toxins, undigested food particles, and bacteria to pass through, leading to inflammation and other health issues.

Factors Affecting Gut Lining Integrity:

- Diet: Consuming a diet high in processed foods, sugar, unhealthy fats, and lacking in nutrients can contribute to gut lining damage and inflammation.
- Chronic Stress: Prolonged stress can negatively impact gut integrity by affecting the gut-brain axis and disrupting the balance of gut bacteria.
- Medications: Certain medications, such as nonsteroidal anti-inflammatory drugs (NSAIDs),

antibiotics, and proton pump inhibitors (PPIs), can damage the gut lining and impair its ability to heal.

- Dysbiosis: An imbalance in the gut microbiota, characterized by an overgrowth of harmful bacteria or a lack of beneficial bacteria, can contribute to gut lining damage.

Strategies for Restoring Gut Integrity:

- Anti-Inflammatory Diet: Adopt an anti-inflammatory diet that focuses on whole, unprocessed foods, rich in antioxidants, fiber, and healthy fats. This diet supports gut healing and reduces inflammation, allowing the gut lining to repair.
- Gut-Healing Foods: Incorporate specific foods that promote gut healing, such as bone broth, collagen, gelatin, and glutamine. These foods provide essential nutrients and support the repair of the gut lining.
- Nutrient Supplementation: Certain nutrients, such as zinc, vitamin A, vitamin D, and omega-3 fatty acids, play a vital role in maintaining gut lining integrity. Consider supplementation under the guidance of a healthcare professional to ensure adequate levels of these nutrients.
- Probiotics and Prebiotics: Probiotics help restore the balance of beneficial gut bacteria, supporting gut health and promoting gut lining repair. Prebiotics, on the other hand, provide nourishment for the beneficial bacteria. Incorporate probiotic-rich foods and prebiotic-rich foods into your diet or consider high-quality supplements.
- Gut-Supportive Herbs and Supplements: Several herbs and supplements have been shown to support gut healing and repair, including slippery elm, aloe vera, licorice root, and marshmallow root. These can be taken in various forms, such as teas, capsules, or powders.
- Reduce Stress: Implement stress-management techniques such as meditation, deep breathing exercises, and regular physical activity. Stress reduction

supports gut healing and the restoration of gut lining
integrity.
•   Identify and Address Food Sensitivities: Work
with a healthcare professional or registered dietitian to
identify and eliminate any food sensitivities that may
contribute to gut lining damage and inflammation.

Restoring gut integrity is essential for overall gut health and
well-being. By implementing strategies such as an anti-
inflammatory diet, incorporating gut-healing foods and
supplements, supporting the gut microbiota, and reducing
stress, we can promote the repair of the gut lining and
reduce inflammation. Healing the gut lining requires a
holistic approach that addresses both the underlying causes
and supports the body's natural healing processes. In the
next chapters, we will continue our exploration of healing
the gut and nurturing optimal health.

3.4 Gut Healing Diets: Exploring Therapeutic Approaches

Diet plays a vital role in gut health and the healing of various
gut-related conditions, including leaky gut syndrome and
gut inflammation. In this chapter, "Gut Healing Diets:
Exploring Therapeutic Approaches," we delve into different
dietary approaches that have shown promise in promoting
gut healing and restoring optimal gut function. By
understanding these therapeutic diets and their
mechanisms of action, individuals can make informed
choices to support their gut health journey.
•   The Specific Carbohydrate Diet (SCD):
The Specific Carbohydrate Diet is a dietary approach that
restricts certain carbohydrates, including grains, lactose,
and complex sugars. The goal of this diet is to starve
harmful gut bacteria and yeasts while promoting the growth
of beneficial bacteria. By reducing inflammation and
restoring gut balance, the SCD can support gut healing and

improve symptoms associated with conditions like Crohn's disease and ulcerative colitis.

• The Low FODMAP Diet:

The Low FODMAP (Fermentable Oligosaccharides, Disaccharides, Monosaccharides, and Polyols) Diet is designed to reduce the consumption of specific types of carbohydrates that can be poorly absorbed and fermented in the gut. This diet has shown effectiveness in managing symptoms of irritable bowel syndrome (IBS), including bloating, gas, and abdominal pain. It provides relief by reducing the intake of fermentable carbohydrates, which can trigger gut symptoms in susceptible individuals.

• The GAPS Diet:

The Gut and Psychology Syndrome (GAPS) Diet focuses on the connection between the gut and mental health. It eliminates processed foods, grains, and sugars while emphasizing nutrient-dense foods, bone broth, fermented foods, and probiotics. The GAPS Diet aims to heal the gut, reduce inflammation, and support mental well-being by addressing conditions such as autism, attention deficit hyperactivity disorder (ADHD), and depression that are believed to be influenced by gut health.

• The Autoimmune Protocol (AIP) Diet:

The Autoimmune Protocol Diet is an elimination diet that removes potential inflammatory foods and triggers, including grains, legumes, dairy, processed sugars, and nightshade vegetables. It is designed to reduce inflammation, support gut healing, and alleviate symptoms associated with autoimmune diseases. By removing foods that can contribute to gut permeability and inflammation, the AIP Diet aims to restore immune balance and promote overall health.

• The Mediterranean Diet:

The Mediterranean Diet is a dietary pattern characterized by a high consumption of fruits, vegetables, whole grains, legumes, lean proteins, and healthy fats such as olive oil and fatty fish. This diet has been associated with numerous health benefits, including improved gut health. Its emphasis on whole, unprocessed foods provides essential nutrients, antioxidants, and fiber, supporting a healthy gut microbiota and reducing inflammation.

- The Elimination Diet:

The Elimination Diet involves temporarily removing potential trigger foods, such as gluten, dairy, soy, eggs, and nuts, from the diet and then reintroducing them one at a time to identify specific food sensitivities. This diet is highly individualized and can help pinpoint foods that may be contributing to gut inflammation, allowing individuals to make personalized dietary adjustments to support gut healing.

- Personalized Nutrition and Gut Healing:

It is important to note that while these therapeutic diets can be beneficial, everyone's gut is unique, and individual responses may vary. Personalized nutrition, based on careful observation and guidance from healthcare professionals or registered dietitians, can provide tailored approaches to address specific gut health issues. This may involve combining elements from different therapeutic diets or incorporating additional gut-healing strategies.

Gut healing diets offer valuable approaches to support gut health, reduce inflammation, and promote overall well-being. By exploring therapeutic dietary approaches such as the Specific Carbohydrate Diet, the Low FODMAP Diet, the GAPS Diet, the Autoimmune Protocol Diet, the Mediterranean Diet, the Elimination Diet, and personalized nutrition, individuals can make informed choices to nourish their gut, promote healing, and alleviate symptoms associated with gut-related conditions. It is essential to consult with healthcare professionals or registered dietitians to ensure these dietary approaches are suitable for individual needs and goals. In the next chapters, we will continue our exploration of healing the gut and nurturing optimal health.

Chapter 3.5: Herbs and Supplements for Gut Health

In addition to dietary changes, herbs and supplements can play a significant role in promoting gut health and supporting gut healing. In this chapter, "Herbs and Supplements for Gut Health," we will explore a variety of natural remedies that have shown potential in improving gut function, reducing inflammation, and supporting the gut microbiota. By understanding the benefits and mechanisms of action of these herbs and supplements, individuals can make informed decisions about incorporating them into their gut health regimen.

- Probiotics:

Probiotics are live beneficial bacteria that can restore and balance the gut microbiota. They are available in various strains, including Lactobacillus and Bifidobacterium, and can be consumed through foods or supplements. Probiotics promote gut health by inhibiting the growth of harmful bacteria, improving gut barrier function, and modulating immune response.

- Digestive Enzymes:

Digestive enzymes are substances that help break down food into smaller molecules for better absorption. They can be particularly beneficial for individuals with digestive disorders or those who have difficulty digesting certain foods. Common digestive enzymes include amylase, protease, and lipase, which aid in the breakdown of carbohydrates, proteins, and fats, respectively.

- Slippery Elm:

Slippery elm is an herb derived from the inner bark of the slippery elm tree. It contains mucilage, a substance that becomes gel-like when mixed with water. This mucilage coats and soothes the lining of the digestive tract, providing relief from inflammation and irritation. Slippery elm can be consumed in the form of tea or capsules.

- Marshmallow Root:

Marshmallow root is known for its demulcent and anti-inflammatory properties. It forms a protective layer along the digestive tract, reducing irritation and promoting healing. Marshmallow root can be consumed as a tea or in supplement form.

- Aloe Vera:

Aloe vera has long been used for its healing properties, including its ability to soothe and repair the gut lining. It contains compounds such as polysaccharides and anthraquinones that possess anti-inflammatory and immune-modulating effects. Aloe vera gel or juice can be consumed internally to support gut health.

- Turmeric:

Turmeric is a spice known for its vibrant yellow color and its active compound, curcumin. Curcumin has powerful anti-inflammatory and antioxidant properties, making it beneficial for gut health. It can help reduce inflammation, support gut barrier function, and modulate the gut microbiota. Turmeric can be used in cooking or taken in supplement form.

- Ginger:

Ginger is a well-known spice with anti-inflammatory and digestive properties. It can help reduce inflammation in the gut, alleviate digestive discomfort, and stimulate digestion. Ginger can be consumed fresh, as a tea, or in supplement form.

- Glutamine:

Glutamine is an amino acid that plays a crucial role in maintaining the integrity of the gut lining. It serves as a fuel source for the cells of the intestinal lining and supports their repair and regeneration. Glutamine can be obtained through dietary sources or taken as a supplement.

- Omega-3 Fatty Acids:

Omega-3 fatty acids, found in fatty fish, flaxseeds, chia seeds, and walnuts, have anti-inflammatory properties that can benefit gut health. They can help reduce gut inflammation, support gut barrier function, and promote a healthy gut microbiota. Omega-3 fatty acids can be obtained through dietary sources or taken as a supplement.

- Zinc:

Zinc is a mineral that plays a vital role in gut health and immune function. It is involved in the maintenance of the gut barrier and supports the regeneration of the gut lining. Zinc can be obtained through dietary sources like oysters, beef, and pumpkin seeds or taken as a supplement.

Herbs and supplements can be valuable additions to a gut health regimen, providing support for gut healing, reducing inflammation, and promoting a healthy gut microbiota. Probiotics, digestive enzymes, slippery elm, marshmallow root, aloe vera, turmeric, ginger, glutamine, omega-3 fatty acids, and zinc are just a few examples of the many natural remedies available. It is important to consult with healthcare professionals or qualified practitioners to determine the appropriate herbs and supplements for individual needs and to ensure safety and efficacy. In the next chapters, we will continue our exploration of healing the gut and nurturing optimal health.

Chapter 4

The Gut-Mind Connection

4.1 Gut Health and Mental Well-being

In recent years, there has been a growing recognition of the intricate relationship between the gut and the mind. The gut-mind connection refers to the bidirectional communication between the gut and the brain, highlighting how the health of our gut can influence our mental well-being and vice versa. In this chapter, "Gut Health and Mental Well-being," we will explore the fascinating link between the gut and mental health, examining the scientific evidence and understanding how nurturing a healthy gut can positively impact our emotional and psychological state.

- The Gut-Brain Axis:

The gut-brain axis is the network of communication pathways between the gut and the brain. It involves various components, including the central nervous system, the enteric nervous system (ENS) within the gut, and the gut microbiota. Signals travel back and forth through these pathways, influencing mood, behavior, and cognitive function. Dysfunction in the gut-brain axis has been associated with conditions such as anxiety, depression, and even neurodegenerative diseases.

- The Role of the Gut Microbiota:

The gut microbiota, the collection of microorganisms residing in our digestive tract, plays a crucial role in the gut-brain axis. These microorganisms communicate with the brain through various mechanisms, including the production of neurotransmitters, such as serotonin and dopamine, and the modulation of immune and inflammatory responses.

Imbalances in the gut microbiota, known as dysbiosis, have been linked to mental health disorders.
- Serotonin and the Gut:
Serotonin, often referred to as the "feel-good" neurotransmitter, is primarily produced in the gut. It influences mood, appetite, and sleep, among other functions. The gut microbiota plays a crucial role in serotonin production, and disruptions in the gut microbial balance can impact serotonin levels, potentially contributing to mood disorders.
- Inflammation and Mental Health:
Chronic inflammation in the gut can have far-reaching effects on mental health. Inflammatory molecules can cross the blood-brain barrier and trigger immune responses in the brain, leading to neuroinflammation. This neuroinflammation has been implicated in the development of depression, anxiety, and cognitive decline. Nurturing a healthy gut and reducing gut inflammation can have positive effects on mental well-being.
- Gut Health and Stress:
The gut-brain axis is closely intertwined with the stress response system. Chronic stress can disrupt the balance of the gut microbiota, impair gut barrier function, and increase inflammation in the gut. This, in turn, can negatively impact mental health. Managing stress and adopting gut-healthy practices can help support a balanced gut-brain axis and promote resilience to stress.
- Nutrition, Gut Health, and Mental Well-being:
Nutrition plays a critical role in supporting both gut health and mental well-being. A diet rich in whole foods, including fruits, vegetables, whole grains, lean proteins, and healthy fats, can provide the necessary nutrients for a healthy gut microbiota and optimal brain function. On the other hand, a diet high in processed foods, sugar, and unhealthy fats can disrupt the gut microbiota and contribute to mental health imbalances.
- Probiotics and Mental Health:

Probiotics, beneficial bacteria that promote gut health, have shown promise in improving mental well-being. Certain strains of probiotics, such as Lactobacillus and Bifidobacterium, have been associated with reduced symptoms of anxiety, depression, and stress. Consuming probiotic-rich foods or taking probiotic supplements can help support a healthy gut microbiota and potentially benefit mental health.

•   Lifestyle Factors for Gut-Mind Balance:
In addition to nutrition and probiotics, other lifestyle factors can contribute to a balanced gut-mind connection. Regular exercise, quality sleep, stress management techniques, and social connections all play roles in supporting gut health and mental well-being. Incorporating these lifestyle practices into daily life can help nurture a healthy gut and promote positive mental health.

The gut-mind connection highlights the importance of nurturing a healthy gut for optimal mental well-being. The gut-brain axis, the gut microbiota, serotonin production, inflammation, stress, nutrition, and probiotics all play integral roles in this complex relationship. By understanding and addressing the factors that influence the gut-mind connection, individuals can take proactive steps to improve their mental health and overall well-being. In the following chapters, we will continue our exploration of the gut-mind connection and delve deeper into strategies for nurturing a healthy gut and supporting mental well-being.

4.2 Stress, Anxiety, and Gut Health

Stress and anxiety are prevalent in today's fast-paced world, affecting millions of people worldwide. While these conditions are often associated with mental health, emerging research suggests that they are closely linked to gut health as well. In this chapter, "Stress, Anxiety, and Gut Health," we will explore the intricate relationship between stress, anxiety, and the gut, examining how stress and anxiety impact gut health and vice versa. By understanding this connection, we can develop strategies to support our gut and manage stress and anxiety effectively.

- The Stress Response and the Gut:

The stress response, also known as the "fight-or-flight" response, triggers a series of physiological changes in the body. During times of stress, the body releases stress hormones such as cortisol, which can impact gut health. Increased cortisol levels can affect gut motility, disrupt the gut microbiota, compromise gut barrier function, and contribute to inflammation.

- Gut-Brain Communication in Stress and Anxiety:

The gut and the brain constantly communicate through the gut-brain axis, allowing bidirectional signaling. Stress and anxiety can alter this communication, leading to changes in gut function and microbial composition. The gut microbiota can also produce molecules that influence brain function and emotional well-being, highlighting the crucial role of gut health in stress and anxiety management.

- The Impact of Stress and Anxiety on Gut Health:

Chronic stress and anxiety can have detrimental effects on gut health. They can increase gut permeability, disrupt the balance of the gut microbiota, impair digestive function, and contribute to gastrointestinal disorders such as irritable bowel syndrome (IBS). Additionally, stress and anxiety can exacerbate gut inflammation and contribute to the development of inflammatory bowel diseases (IBD).

- Gut Microbiota and Stress:

The gut microbiota plays a pivotal role in the stress response. Research has shown that the composition of the gut microbiota can influence how individuals respond to stress and anxiety. Imbalances in the gut microbiota, such as reduced microbial diversity or an overgrowth of harmful bacteria, have been associated with increased susceptibility to stress and anxiety disorders.

- Strategies for Managing Stress and Anxiety to Support Gut Health:

Managing stress and anxiety is essential for maintaining a healthy gut. Various strategies can be employed to support gut health while managing these conditions. These include stress reduction techniques such as mindfulness meditation, deep breathing exercises, regular physical activity, and adequate sleep. Additionally, incorporating relaxation practices like yoga, massage, and aromatherapy can help promote a healthy gut-brain axis.

- Diet and Gut Health in Stress and Anxiety Management:

Nutrition plays a significant role in managing stress and anxiety while supporting gut health. Consuming a balanced diet rich in whole foods, including fruits, vegetables, whole grains, lean proteins, and healthy fats, provides the necessary nutrients for optimal gut function and supports the body's stress response system. Avoiding processed foods, caffeine, and excessive sugar can also help maintain gut health and manage stress and anxiety.

- Probiotics and Gut-Brain Connection:

Probiotics, beneficial bacteria that support gut health, have shown promising effects on stress and anxiety management. Certain strains of probiotics, such as Lactobacillus and Bifidobacterium, have been associated with reduced symptoms of stress and anxiety. Consuming probiotic-rich foods like yogurt, kefir, and sauerkraut or taking probiotic supplements can help restore gut microbial balance and potentially alleviate stress and anxiety symptoms.

- Seeking Professional Support:

For individuals experiencing chronic stress and anxiety, seeking professional support is crucial. Mental health professionals can provide guidance and therapeutic interventions tailored to individual needs. Additionally, consulting with a registered dietitian or healthcare practitioner who specializes in gut health can offer personalized dietary recommendations and support for managing stress and anxiety while prioritizing gut health.

Conclusion:

The interplay between stress, anxiety, and gut health is a complex and fascinating area of research. Chronic stress and anxiety can significantly impact gut health, while nurturing a healthy gut can help manage these conditions. By understanding the relationship between stress, anxiety, and the gut, individuals can implement strategies such as stress reduction techniques, a gut-healthy diet, and probiotic supplementation to support their gut health and overall well-being. In the subsequent chapters, we will further explore the connection between gut health and various aspects of our lives, providing insights and practical tips for nurturing a thriving gut.

4.3 Gut Health Strategies for Improved Sleep

Sleep is a vital component of overall health and well-being. It plays a crucial role in physical and mental restoration, immune function, and cognitive performance. Surprisingly, the health of our gut can significantly impact the quality of our sleep. In this chapter, "Gut Health Strategies for Improved Sleep," we will explore the connection between gut health and sleep, understanding how nurturing a healthy gut can positively influence our sleep patterns. We will also discuss practical strategies to optimize gut health and promote restful, rejuvenating sleep.
- The Gut-Sleep Connection:
The gut and sleep have a bidirectional relationship. Disruptions in gut health, such as gut dysbiosis or inflammation, can affect sleep quality and duration. On the other hand, poor sleep can impact gut health by altering gut microbiota composition, increasing gut permeability, and contributing to gastrointestinal symptoms.
- Gut Microbiota and Sleep:
Emerging research suggests that the gut microbiota plays a crucial role in regulating sleep patterns. The gut microbiota produces neurotransmitters and metabolites that influence sleep, such as serotonin, melatonin, and short-chain fatty acids. Imbalances in the gut microbiota composition have

been linked to sleep disorders, including insomnia and sleep apnea.

• Gut Inflammation and Sleep:
Inflammation in the gut can have a negative impact on sleep. Chronic gut inflammation can disrupt sleep patterns, impair sleep quality, and contribute to sleep disorders. Addressing gut inflammation through dietary and lifestyle modifications can help restore a healthy sleep-wake cycle.

• The Role of Diet in Sleep:
Nutrition plays a vital role in supporting both gut health and sleep. Certain dietary factors can either promote or hinder sleep quality. We will explore foods that support a healthy gut and aid in sleep regulation, including those rich in tryptophan, magnesium, and B vitamins. Additionally, we will discuss the importance of meal timing and avoiding foods that can disrupt sleep, such as caffeine and heavy, greasy meals.

• Fiber and Sleep:
Dietary fiber is essential for gut health and can also influence sleep. Fiber-rich foods, such as fruits, vegetables, whole grains, and legumes, support a diverse and healthy gut microbiota. Additionally, fiber can help regulate blood sugar levels, promoting stable energy levels throughout the day and a more restful sleep at night.

• Probiotics and Sleep:
Probiotics, beneficial bacteria that support gut health, have shown promise in improving sleep quality. Certain strains of probiotics, such as Lactobacillus and Bifidobacterium, have been associated with better sleep outcomes. Consuming probiotic-rich foods or taking probiotic supplements can help optimize gut health and potentially enhance sleep.

• Sleep Hygiene and Gut Health:
Good sleep hygiene practices contribute to both sleep quality and gut health. We will discuss strategies to create a sleep-friendly environment, establish a consistent sleep routine, and manage stress before bed. These practices can help synchronize the body's natural circadian rhythm and support optimal gut function.

•	Lifestyle Factors for Restful Sleep:
In addition to diet and sleep hygiene, certain lifestyle factors can promote restful sleep and gut health. Regular exercise, stress management techniques, limiting electronic device use before bed, and creating a calm bedtime routine all contribute to improved sleep quality and a healthy gut.
Conclusion:
Nurturing a healthy gut can have a profound impact on sleep quality and overall well-being. The gut-sleep connection highlights the importance of adopting strategies that support gut health to optimize sleep. By implementing gut-friendly dietary choices, incorporating probiotics, practicing good sleep hygiene, and embracing a healthy lifestyle, individuals can improve their sleep patterns and wake up feeling refreshed and rejuvenated. In the following chapters, we will continue to explore the multifaceted relationship between gut health and various aspects of our lives, providing insights and practical guidance for nurturing a thriving gut and enhancing overall health.

4.4 Mindful Eating: Nourishing Your Gut and Mind

In today's fast-paced world, we often find ourselves rushing through meals, eating on the go, and mindlessly consuming food without paying attention to our bodies and the nourishment it needs. However, adopting a mindful eating practice can not only support our gut health but also enhance our overall well-being. In this chapter, "Mindful Eating: Nourishing Your Gut and Mind," we will explore the concept of mindful eating, its benefits for gut health, and practical strategies to incorporate mindful eating into our daily lives.
•	Understanding Mindful Eating:
Mindful eating is the practice of bringing our full attention and awareness to the present moment when eating. It involves engaging all our senses, observing our thoughts and emotions around food, and cultivating a non-judgmental attitude towards our eating experiences. Mindful

eating encourages us to savor the flavors, textures, and aromas of our food, fostering a deeper connection with the act of eating.
•	The Gut-Mind Connection in Mindful Eating: Mindful eating has a profound impact on the gut-mind connection. By slowing down and being fully present during meals, we can activate the rest-and-digest response of the autonomic nervous system, promoting optimal digestion and nutrient absorption. Mindful eating also helps reduce stress levels, which can positively influence gut health by decreasing inflammation and supporting a balanced gut microbiota.
•	Benefits of Mindful Eating for Gut Health: Practicing mindful eating offers several benefits for gut health. It aids in proper digestion, reducing the likelihood of gastrointestinal issues such as bloating, indigestion, and acid reflux. Mindful eating promotes a healthy relationship with food, preventing overeating and promoting better portion control. It also enhances our ability to recognize hunger and satiety cues, supporting a balanced and nourished gut.
•	Cultivating Mindful Eating Habits: Incorporating mindful eating habits into our daily lives requires intention and practice. We will explore practical strategies to cultivate mindful eating habits, such as setting a calm and inviting eating environment, practicing mindful breathing before meals, chewing food thoroughly, and taking breaks between bites to savor the flavors. We will also discuss the importance of tuning in to hunger and fullness cues, as well as identifying emotional and non-hunger triggers for eating.
•	The Role of Mindful Eating in Food Choices: Mindful eating extends beyond the act of eating itself. It also influences our food choices and preferences. By being present and attuned to our bodies, we can make conscious decisions about the foods we consume, prioritizing those that nourish our gut and overall health. We will explore how mindful eating helps us become more attuned to our body's

needs and develop a deeper appreciation for whole, nutrient-dense foods.

• Mindful Eating and Emotional Well-being:
Our emotions and mental state often impact our relationship with food. Mindful eating can help us develop a healthier relationship with food by fostering awareness of emotional eating patterns and promoting self-compassion. We will discuss strategies to navigate emotional eating through mindful awareness and alternative coping mechanisms that nurture both our gut and emotional well-being.

• Mindful Eating and Sustainable Food Choices:
In addition to benefiting our gut health, mindful eating encourages us to consider the environmental impact of our food choices. We will explore how mindfulness can extend to making sustainable and ethical food choices, such as opting for locally sourced, organic produce and reducing food waste.

• Mindful Eating as a Lifestyle Practice:
Mindful eating is not a quick fix or a temporary diet. It is a lifelong practice that can transform our relationship with food and support our gut health and overall well-being. We will discuss strategies to integrate mindful eating into our daily lives, create mindful eating rituals, and navigate challenging situations where mindless eating is prevalent.

Conclusion:
Mindful eating is a powerful practice that nourishes both our gut and mind. By bringing awareness, intention, and presence to our meals, we can enhance our digestion, support a healthy gut microbiota, and develop a balanced and joyful relationship with food. As we continue our journey through this book, we will explore further the intricate connections between gut health and different aspects of our lives, offering guidance for nurturing a harmonious gut and fostering optimal well-being.

4.5 Gut Health and Emotional Balance

Emotions and gut health are deeply intertwined, forming a complex connection that influences our overall well-being. In this chapter, "Gut Health and Emotional Balance," we will explore the relationship between gut health and emotions, understanding how nurturing a healthy gut can positively impact our emotional balance. We will delve into the science behind this connection and discuss practical strategies to support both gut health and emotional well-being.
- The Gut-Emotion Connection:
The gut is often referred to as our "second brain" due to its extensive network of neurons and neurotransmitters. This gut-brain connection, known as the gut-brain axis, allows bidirectional communication between the gut and the brain, affecting our emotions, mood, and mental health. We will explore how the gut influences emotional processes and how emotions, in turn, impact gut health.
- Gut Health and Serotonin:
Serotonin, often referred to as the "feel-good" neurotransmitter, is primarily produced in the gut. A healthy gut microbiota is crucial for maintaining optimal serotonin levels, which play a significant role in regulating mood and emotions. We will discuss how imbalances in the gut microbiota can disrupt serotonin production and contribute to emotional imbalances.
- Gut Inflammation and Emotional Well-being:
Chronic gut inflammation can have a detrimental impact on emotional well-being. Inflammation in the gut can trigger an immune response that can affect brain function and contribute to symptoms of anxiety and depression. We will explore the mechanisms behind gut inflammation and its role in emotional disturbances.
- Gut Microbiota and Emotional Health:
The composition of the gut microbiota plays a vital role in emotional balance. Imbalances in the gut microbiota, known as dysbiosis, have been associated with various mental health conditions, including anxiety and depression. We will

discuss how nurturing a diverse and balanced gut microbiota through diet, probiotics, and other lifestyle factors can support emotional well-being.
•	Stress, Gut Health, and Emotions:
Stress is a significant factor that influences both gut health and emotions. Chronic stress can disrupt the gut microbiota, increase gut permeability, and lead to inflammation, impacting emotional balance. We will explore strategies to manage stress and cultivate resilience, supporting both gut health and emotional well-being.
•	Mind-Body Practices for Gut-Emotion Balance:
Mind-body practices such as meditation, yoga, and deep breathing techniques can play a significant role in promoting emotional balance and gut health. These practices have been shown to reduce stress, improve gut function, and enhance emotional well-being. We will discuss the benefits of these practices and how to incorporate them into our daily lives.
•	Nutrition for Emotional Well-being:
Nutrition plays a vital role in supporting both gut health and emotional balance. We will explore specific nutrients and dietary patterns that can positively influence emotions, such as omega-3 fatty acids, B vitamins, and a whole foods-based diet. We will also discuss the importance of mindful eating and its impact on emotional well-being.
•	Gut-Healing Strategies for Emotional Balance:
Addressing gut health is essential for promoting emotional balance. We will discuss gut-healing strategies, including dietary modifications, probiotics, lifestyle changes, and gut-supporting supplements. These approaches aim to reduce inflammation, restore gut microbiota balance, and support optimal gut function, ultimately contributing to improved emotional well-being.

Nurturing a healthy gut is crucial for supporting emotional balance and overall well-being. The intricate relationship between gut health and emotions highlights the importance of addressing gut health to promote emotional well-being.

By implementing strategies to support gut health, managing stress, practicing mind-body techniques, and adopting a nourishing diet, we can cultivate a harmonious gut-emotion connection and enhance our emotional balance for a fulfilling and vibrant life.

Chapter 5

Lifestyle Factors for a Healthy Gut

5.1 Exercise and Gut Health: Moving Toward Balance

Regular physical exercise is well-known for its numerous benefits on overall health and well-being. However, its impact on gut health is often overlooked. In this chapter, "Exercise and Gut Health: Moving Toward Balance," we will explore the connection between exercise and the gut, understanding how physical activity can support a healthy gut. We will delve into the mechanisms behind this relationship and discuss practical strategies to incorporate exercise into our lifestyle for optimal gut health.

- The Gut-Exercise Connection:
Exercise influences the gut in various ways, impacting gut motility, microbial diversity, and overall gut function. We will explore the mechanisms behind this connection, including the role of exercise in promoting gut peristalsis, enhancing blood flow to the gut, and modulating the gut microbiota.

- Exercise and Gut Motility:
Regular exercise has been shown to improve gut motility, aiding in the movement of food through the digestive system. We will discuss how exercise stimulates the contraction and relaxation of intestinal muscles, promoting regular bowel movements and preventing issues such as constipation.

- Exercise and Gut Microbiota:
Physical activity plays a significant role in shaping the composition and diversity of the gut microbiota. We will explore how exercise influences the gut microbial community, promoting the growth of beneficial bacteria and enhancing microbial richness. Additionally, we will discuss

the potential implications of exercise-induced changes in the gut microbiota for overall gut health.
•	Gut Permeability and Exercise:
Exercise has been found to modulate gut permeability, also known as "leaky gut." We will explore how regular physical activity can help maintain the integrity of the gut lining, reducing the passage of harmful substances into the bloodstream. We will also discuss the potential impact of exercise on reducing gut inflammation and its role in preventing conditions associated with increased gut permeability.
•	Exercise Intensity and Gut Health:
The intensity of exercise can influence its impact on gut health. We will explore the relationship between exercise intensity and gut function, discussing how moderate-intensity exercise may be particularly beneficial for gut health. We will also discuss considerations for individuals engaging in high-intensity exercise and the importance of balancing exercise with adequate recovery for optimal gut health.
•	Practical Strategies for Incorporating Exercise:
We will discuss practical strategies for incorporating exercise into our daily lives to support gut health. This includes finding activities that we enjoy, setting realistic goals, and creating a consistent exercise routine. We will explore different types of exercise, including aerobic activities, strength training, and mind-body practices, and discuss their potential benefits for gut health.
•	Timing of Exercise and Gut Function:
The timing of exercise in relation to meals can impact gut function. We will discuss the effects of pre-exercise and post-exercise nutrition on gut health and provide guidelines for optimizing the timing of meals and snacks to support digestion and gut function.
•	Supporting Gut Health during Exercise:
Proper hydration and nutrition during exercise are essential for supporting gut health. We will discuss strategies for maintaining hydration, fueling the body with appropriate

nutrients, and avoiding common gastrointestinal issues that may arise during exercise. We will also explore the role of probiotics and gut-supporting supplements in supporting gut health during exercise.

Incorporating regular exercise into our lifestyle not only benefits our overall health but also supports a healthy gut. By understanding the gut-exercise connection and implementing practical strategies for incorporating physical activity into our daily lives, we can optimize gut motility, enhance gut microbial diversity, and promote gut health. By prioritizing exercise as a lifestyle factor for a healthy gut, we can move toward a balanced and thriving digestive system.

5.2: Sleep and Circadian Rhythms: Resetting Your Gut Clock

Sleep is a fundamental aspect of our well-being, and its impact extends beyond just feeling rested. In this chapter, "Sleep and Circadian Rhythms: Resetting Your Gut Clock," we will explore the profound connection between sleep, circadian rhythms, and gut health. We will delve into the importance of sleep for maintaining a healthy gut, understanding the role of circadian rhythms in gut function, and discussing practical strategies to optimize sleep for optimal gut health.

- The Sleep-Gut Connection:

Sleep and gut health are intricately intertwined, forming a bidirectional relationship. We will explore how sleep disturbances can negatively impact gut health, contributing to issues such as gut inflammation, altered gut microbiota, and impaired gut motility. Additionally, we will discuss how an unhealthy gut can disrupt sleep patterns, creating a cycle of sleep-gut dysfunction.

- Circadian Rhythms and Gut Function:

Circadian rhythms, the internal biological clocks that regulate various physiological processes, play a crucial role in gut health and function. We will discuss the influence of circadian rhythms on gut motility, gut microbiota composition, and the secretion of digestive enzymes and hormones. Understanding the importance of aligning our daily routines with our circadian rhythms can help optimize gut health.

- Sleep Quality and Gut Health:
Quality sleep is essential for maintaining a healthy gut. We will explore the impact of sleep duration, sleep efficiency, and sleep stages on gut health. We will discuss the role of rapid eye movement (REM) sleep and non-rapid eye movement (NREM) sleep in promoting gut restoration and repair processes. We will also address common sleep disorders and their implications for gut health.

- Gut Health Strategies for Improved Sleep:
Supporting gut health can positively impact sleep quality. We will discuss specific gut health strategies, including dietary modifications, probiotics, and lifestyle changes, that can improve sleep. By addressing gut imbalances, reducing gut inflammation, and supporting a healthy gut microbiota, we can create an environment conducive to restful and rejuvenating sleep.

- The Gut Clock and Meal Timing:
The timing of meals and fasting periods can influence our gut clock and overall gut health. We will explore the concept of time-restricted eating and discuss the benefits of aligning our meal timing with our circadian rhythms. We will also delve into the impact of irregular meal schedules, late-night eating, and shift work on gut health and sleep patterns.

- Creating a Sleep-Optimized Environment:
Creating a sleep-friendly environment is essential for promoting quality sleep and optimal gut health. We will discuss practical strategies to optimize our sleep environment, including optimizing bedroom conditions, establishing a bedtime routine, and reducing exposure to electronic devices and artificial light that can disrupt our natural sleep-wake cycles.

- Sleep Hygiene Practices for Gut Health:
Implementing healthy sleep hygiene practices is crucial for resetting our gut clock and promoting gut health. We will

discuss strategies for improving sleep hygiene, such as maintaining a consistent sleep schedule, practicing relaxation techniques before bed, and managing stress levels. These practices help synchronize our circadian rhythms and promote healthy sleep patterns.
- The Role of Melatonin in Gut Health: Melatonin, a hormone primarily associated with regulating sleep-wake cycles, also plays a role in gut health. We will explore how melatonin influences gut function, including its antioxidant and anti-inflammatory properties. We will discuss natural ways to support melatonin production and its potential benefits for gut health.

Sleep and circadian rhythms are integral to maintaining a healthy gut. By recognizing the intricate relationship between sleep, gut health, and circadian rhythms, and implementing practical strategies to optimize sleep, we can reset our gut clock and support optimal gut function. Prioritizing quality sleep as a lifestyle factor for a healthy gut allows us to create a harmonious balance between rest, rejuvenation, and gut well-being.

5.3 Gut Health and Stress Management Techniques

Stress has a profound impact on our overall well-being, and its effects extend to the health of our gut. In this chapter, "Gut Health and Stress Management Techniques," we will explore the intricate relationship between stress and gut health, understanding how chronic stress can disrupt gut function and contribute to digestive issues. We will delve into various stress management techniques and discuss their potential benefits in promoting a healthy gut.
- The Stress-Gut Connection: Stress triggers a cascade of physiological responses in our body, including those that directly impact the gut. We will explore how chronic stress can lead to increased gut permeability, alterations in gut microbiota composition, and changes in gut motility. Understanding the stress-gut

connection is essential for implementing effective stress management techniques.

* Stress, Gut Microbiota, and Gut-Brain Axis: The gut microbiota and the gut-brain axis play a crucial role in mediating the impact of stress on gut health. We will discuss how stress can influence the composition and diversity of gut microbiota, affecting gut function and overall well-being. Additionally, we will explore the bidirectional communication between the gut and the brain and its implications for stress-related gut issues.
* Mind-Body Techniques for Stress Management: Various mind-body techniques have been shown to effectively reduce stress levels and promote gut health. We will discuss techniques such as mindfulness meditation, deep breathing exercises, yoga, and progressive muscle relaxation. These practices help activate the body's relaxation response, counteracting the physiological effects of stress on the gut.
* Exercise for Stress Reduction and Gut Health: Regular exercise not only benefits the gut but also acts as a potent stress management tool. We will explore how physical activity can help reduce stress levels, promote the release of endorphins, and improve overall well-being. Engaging in exercise that aligns with individual preferences and abilities can effectively alleviate stress and support gut health.
* Nutrition for Stress Reduction and Gut Health: Diet plays a crucial role in managing stress and supporting gut health. We will discuss nutrient-dense foods that promote resilience against stress, including those rich in omega-3 fatty acids, B vitamins, and antioxidants. We will also explore the impact of gut-friendly foods on stress reduction and gut microbiota balance.
* Sleep and Restorative Practices: Adequate sleep and restorative practices are essential for managing stress and promoting gut health. We will discuss the importance of prioritizing sleep, establishing a consistent sleep routine, and creating a conducive sleep

environment. Additionally, we will explore relaxation techniques such as aromatherapy, warm baths, and soothing music that can facilitate stress reduction and support gut health.

- Cognitive-Behavioral Techniques for Stress Management:

Cognitive-behavioral techniques provide valuable tools for managing stress and improving gut health. We will discuss strategies such as cognitive reframing, stress management techniques, and time management skills. These techniques help reframe negative thought patterns, reduce stress levels, and promote a more balanced perspective.

- Social Support and Connection:

Social support and maintaining meaningful connections play a vital role in stress management and gut health. We will explore the importance of nurturing supportive relationships, engaging in positive social interactions, and seeking emotional support when needed. Building a strong support system contributes to resilience against stress and fosters overall well-being.

Conclusion:

Managing stress is crucial for maintaining a healthy gut. By understanding the stress-gut connection and implementing effective stress management techniques, we can reduce the impact of stress on gut function and promote digestive wellness. Mind-body techniques, exercise, nutrition, restorative practices, cognitive-behavioral strategies, and social support all contribute to a comprehensive approach to stress management and gut health. By prioritizing stress reduction, we pave the way for a harmonious gut-brain axis and improved overall well-being.

5.4: Environmental Factors and Gut Health

Our gut health is influenced not only by internal factors but also by various external environmental factors. In this chapter, "Environmental Factors and Gut Health," we will explore the impact of environmental factors on the health and balance of our gut microbiota. We will discuss how elements such as pollution, toxins, antibiotics, and lifestyle choices can affect the delicate ecosystem within our gut, and we will explore strategies to mitigate their negative effects and promote a healthy gut.

- The Gut Microbiota and Environmental Factors: The gut microbiota, composed of trillions of microorganisms, is highly sensitive to environmental influences. We will examine the role of environmental factors, such as pollution, in disrupting the diversity and composition of the gut microbiota. Additionally, we will explore how exposure to toxins and chemicals can compromise gut health and contribute to various digestive issues.

- Air and Water Quality:
Air and water quality play a significant role in gut health. We will discuss the impact of air pollution, including particulate matter and harmful gases, on gut inflammation, dysbiosis, and gut-related disorders. We will also explore the importance of clean and safe drinking water in maintaining a healthy gut microbiota.

- Pesticides, Antibiotics, and Gut Microbiota:
The use of pesticides in agriculture and the overuse of antibiotics have far-reaching consequences for our gut health. We will examine how exposure to pesticides and the consumption of pesticide residues in food can disrupt the gut microbiota. Additionally, we will discuss the importance of responsible antibiotic use and explore strategies to support the restoration of a healthy gut microbiota after antibiotic treatment.

- Food Additives and Gut Health:
Food additives, including artificial sweeteners, preservatives, and emulsifiers, can have detrimental effects on gut health. We will explore how these additives can disrupt the gut microbiota, increase gut permeability, and contribute to digestive issues. We will discuss the importance of reading labels, making informed food

choices, and opting for whole, unprocessed foods to support a healthy gut.

- Lifestyle Factors and Gut Health:

Various lifestyle choices can impact our gut health. We will discuss the role of stress, sleep, physical activity, and smoking in gut function and the gut microbiota. Understanding the influence of these lifestyle factors allows us to make informed decisions that promote a healthy gut environment.

- Gut Health and Outdoor Spaces:

Spending time in nature and green spaces can positively influence gut health. We will explore the benefits of exposure to natural environments, including increased microbial diversity, reduced stress levels, and improved overall well-being. We will discuss the importance of connecting with nature and incorporating outdoor activities into our daily lives for gut health promotion.

- Gut Health-Friendly Home Environment:

Creating a gut health-friendly home environment involves minimizing exposure to toxins and maintaining good hygiene practices. We will discuss strategies to reduce household toxins, such as using natural cleaning products, filtering tap water, and improving indoor air quality. We will also explore the role of pets and the gut microbiota, emphasizing the importance of maintaining a clean living environment.

- Strategies to Mitigate Environmental Impacts:

Although we cannot completely avoid environmental factors, we can adopt strategies to mitigate their negative effects on gut health. We will discuss practices such as organic food choices, water filtration, and air purifiers that help minimize exposure to harmful substances. Additionally, we will explore the use of probiotics, prebiotics, and dietary fiber to support a resilient gut microbiota in the face of environmental challenges.

Conclusion:

Environmental factors significantly impact our gut health and the delicate balance of our gut microbiota. By understanding the effects of pollution, toxins, antibiotics, and lifestyle choices, we can take proactive steps to mitigate their negative impacts. Creating a gut health-friendly environment involves making conscious choices about our food, water, air, and lifestyle. By prioritizing clean, natural living and adopting strategies to support a healthy gut microbiota, we promote digestive wellness and overall well-being.

5.5 Mind-Body Practices for Gut Harmony

The intricate connection between the mind and the gut is undeniable. In this chapter, "Mind-Body Practices for Gut Harmony," we will explore the powerful influence of our thoughts, emotions, and mental well-being on gut health. We will delve into various mind-body practices and techniques that can help cultivate a harmonious relationship between the mind and the gut, promoting optimal digestive function and overall gut harmony.

- The Gut-Brain Axis and Mind-Body Connection: The gut-brain axis serves as a bidirectional communication system between the gut and the brain. We will discuss how stress, emotions, and mental states can affect gut function through this axis. Understanding this connection is essential for harnessing the power of mind-body practices to promote gut harmony.
- Mindfulness Meditation:
Mindfulness meditation involves focusing one's attention on the present moment with an attitude of non-judgmental awareness. We will explore the benefits of mindfulness meditation in reducing stress, promoting relaxation, and enhancing gut health. Techniques for cultivating mindfulness, such as breath awareness and body scanning, will be discussed.
- Yoga for Digestive Wellness:
Yoga combines physical postures, breath control, and meditation to promote holistic well-being. We will examine specific yoga poses and sequences that target the digestive

system, improving digestion, relieving bloating, and enhancing gut motility. Additionally, we will explore the role of deep breathing exercises (pranayama) in supporting gut health.

- Guided Imagery and Visualization:
Guided imagery and visualization involve using the power of the mind to create positive mental images and experiences. We will discuss how these techniques can be utilized to reduce stress, alleviate gut-related symptoms, and promote overall gut harmony. Guided imagery scripts and visualization exercises will be provided.

- Cognitive-Behavioral Therapy (CBT) for Gut Health:
Cognitive-Behavioral Therapy (CBT) is a psychotherapeutic approach that focuses on identifying and modifying negative thoughts and behaviors. We will explore how CBT techniques can be applied to manage stress, anxiety, and gut-related disorders. Strategies for identifying and reframing negative thoughts will be discussed.

- Relaxation Techniques for Gut Harmony:
Relaxation techniques, such as progressive muscle relaxation, autogenic training, and biofeedback, can induce a state of deep relaxation and alleviate stress-related gut issues. We will explore these techniques and their potential benefits in promoting gut harmony and overall well-being. Practical exercises for relaxation will be provided.

- Journaling for Gut Health:
Keeping a journal can be a valuable tool for self-reflection and emotional expression, contributing to gut health. We will discuss the benefits of journaling in identifying gut triggers, tracking symptoms, and exploring the relationship between emotions and digestive wellness. Prompts and exercises for gut-focused journaling will be shared.

- Expressive Arts Therapies:
Engaging in expressive arts, such as music therapy, art therapy, and dance/movement therapy, can provide a creative outlet for emotional expression and stress

reduction. We will explore how these therapies can positively impact gut health by promoting emotional well-being, self-expression, and relaxation. Suggestions for incorporating expressive arts into daily life will be provided.
•   Laughter Therapy and Humor for Gut Health: Laughter therapy harnesses the healing power of laughter to reduce stress, improve mood, and support gut health. We will discuss the physiological and psychological benefits of laughter and explore ways to incorporate humor into our daily lives for gut harmony.

Mind-body practices offer powerful tools for promoting gut harmony by nurturing the connection between the mind and the gut. By incorporating techniques such as mindfulness meditation, yoga, guided imagery, cognitive-behavioral therapy, relaxation techniques, journaling, expressive arts therapies, and laughter therapy into our lives, we can cultivate a balanced and harmonious gut environment. These practices empower us to manage stress, regulate emotions, and foster a positive mindset, all of which are crucial for optimal digestive function and overall gut health.

Chapter 6

<u>Gut Health and Digestive Disorders</u>

6.1 Irritable Bowel Syndrome (IBS): Understanding and Managing Symptoms

Irritable Bowel Syndrome (IBS) is a common digestive disorder that affects millions of people worldwide. In this chapter, "Irritable Bowel Syndrome (IBS): Understanding and Managing Symptoms," we will delve into the complexities of IBS, exploring its causes, symptoms, and various management strategies. By understanding the underlying mechanisms of IBS and implementing effective coping techniques, individuals can gain control over their symptoms and improve their quality of life.

- What is Irritable Bowel Syndrome (IBS)?

We will begin by defining IBS and discussing its prevalence, demographics, and potential triggers. We will explore the primary symptoms of IBS, including abdominal pain, bloating, altered bowel habits, and their impact on daily life.

- Subtypes of IBS:

IBS can be categorized into subtypes based on predominant bowel habits. We will examine the differences between the subtypes (IBS-D, IBS-C, IBS-M) and how they manifest in terms of symptoms, triggers, and treatment approaches.

- Causes and Triggers of IBS:

The exact causes of IBS remain unclear; however, several factors contribute to its development and symptom exacerbation. We will discuss potential triggers, such as food intolerances, stress, gut dysbiosis, and alterations in gut motility, and their impact on IBS symptoms.

- Diagnostic Process for IBS:

We will explore the diagnostic criteria for IBS, which includes symptom assessment, ruling out other potential causes, and the role of diagnostic tests. We will emphasize the importance of seeking medical evaluation for a proper diagnosis and to rule out other digestive disorders.

- Lifestyle Modifications for Managing IBS Symptoms:

Various lifestyle modifications can help individuals manage their IBS symptoms effectively. We will discuss dietary changes, such as the low FODMAP diet, fiber intake adjustments, and the importance of maintaining regular meal patterns. We will also explore the role of stress management techniques, regular physical activity, and adequate sleep in managing IBS symptoms.

- Medications and Supplements for IBS:

Pharmaceutical interventions and supplements can provide relief for individuals with IBS. We will discuss different medication options, such as antispasmodics, antidepressants, and probiotics, their mechanisms of action, and their potential benefits in managing specific symptoms of IBS.

- Psychological Interventions for IBS:

Given the strong connection between the gut and the brain, psychological interventions play a crucial role in managing IBS symptoms. We will explore cognitive-behavioral therapy (CBT), gut-directed hypnotherapy, and relaxation techniques as effective psychological interventions for reducing stress, improving symptom control, and enhancing overall well-being.

- Complementary and Alternative Therapies for IBS:

Several complementary and alternative therapies show promise in managing IBS symptoms. We will discuss the potential benefits of acupuncture, herbal remedies, probiotics, and mind-body practices such as yoga and meditation. We will provide an overview of the evidence supporting their use in IBS management.

- Coping Strategies for Living with IBS:

Living with IBS can be challenging, both physically and emotionally. We will explore coping strategies to help individuals navigate daily life with IBS, including self-care practices, support networks, and the importance of open communication with healthcare providers.

IBS is a complex digestive disorder that requires a comprehensive approach to symptom management. By understanding the causes, triggers, and available treatment options, individuals with IBS can develop personalized strategies to effectively manage their symptoms and improve their quality of life. It is essential to work closely with healthcare professionals to tailor interventions and find a multifaceted approach that suits each individual's unique needs.

6.2 Inflammatory Bowel Disease (IBD): Strategies for Gut Health

Inflammatory Bowel Disease (IBD) is a chronic condition characterized by inflammation in the digestive tract. This chapter, "Inflammatory Bowel Disease (IBD): Strategies for Gut Health," aims to provide a comprehensive understanding of IBD, including its types, symptoms, underlying mechanisms, and effective strategies for managing the disease. By implementing a holistic approach to gut health, individuals with IBD can minimize symptoms, promote healing, and improve their overall well-being.

- Understanding Inflammatory Bowel Disease (IBD): We will start by defining IBD and differentiating between its two main forms: Crohn's disease and ulcerative colitis. We will explore the underlying causes of IBD, including genetic factors, immune system dysregulation, and environmental triggers.
- Symptoms and Disease Course: We will discuss the common symptoms associated with IBD, such as abdominal pain, diarrhea, rectal bleeding, weight loss, and fatigue. Additionally, we will delve into the

different disease courses and the potential complications that individuals with IBD may face.

- Diagnosis and Medical Management of IBD:
The diagnosis of IBD involves a combination of clinical evaluation, imaging studies, endoscopic procedures, and laboratory tests. We will discuss the importance of early diagnosis and the various medications used to manage IBD, including anti-inflammatory drugs, immunomodulators, and biologic therapies.
- Dietary Approaches for Managing IBD:
Nutrition plays a significant role in managing IBD symptoms and promoting gut healing. We will explore dietary strategies such as the low-residue diet, specific carbohydrate diet (SCD), and the Mediterranean diet, and their potential benefits for individuals with IBD. We will also discuss the importance of personalized nutrition plans and the role of registered dietitians in IBD management.
- Managing Inflammation and Promoting Gut Healing:
Reducing inflammation and promoting gut healing are crucial goals in managing IBD. We will explore lifestyle modifications, including stress reduction techniques, regular exercise, and smoking cessation, that can help minimize inflammation and support the healing process in the gut.
- Medications for Inflammatory Bowel Disease:
We will discuss the different medications used to treat IBD, including aminosalicylates, corticosteroids, immunomodulators, and biologic therapies. We will explore their mechanisms of action, potential side effects, and their role in achieving and maintaining remission in IBD.
- Surgical Interventions for IBD:
In some cases, surgical intervention may be necessary for individuals with IBD. We will discuss the various surgical options, such as bowel resection, ostomy surgery, and colectomy, and their role in managing complications and improving quality of life.
- Complementary and Alternative Therapies for IBD:

Several complementary and alternative therapies can be used alongside conventional treatments to manage IBD symptoms. We will explore the potential benefits of probiotics, omega-3 fatty acids, herbal remedies, acupuncture, and mind-body practices in reducing inflammation, alleviating symptoms, and supporting overall gut health.

• Psychological Support and Coping Strategies: Living with a chronic condition like IBD can have a significant impact on mental health and overall well-being. We will discuss the importance of psychological support, coping strategies, and support networks in managing the emotional challenges that often accompany IBD.
Conclusion:
Managing Inflammatory Bowel Disease requires a comprehensive approach that addresses the underlying inflammation, promotes gut healing, and supports overall well-being. By understanding the disease, implementing appropriate dietary strategies, utilizing medication effectively, considering surgical options when necessary, exploring complementary therapies, and prioritizing psychological support, individuals with IBD can achieve better symptom control, reduce inflammation, and enhance their quality of life. It is crucial to work closely with healthcare professionals to develop a personalized management plan that suits each individual's specific needs.

6.3 Acid Reflux and GERD: Soothing the Flames

Acid reflux and gastroesophageal reflux disease (GERD) are common digestive disorders that can cause discomfort and affect the quality of life. In this chapter, "Acid Reflux and GERD: Soothing the Flames," we will explore the causes, symptoms, and effective strategies for managing these conditions. By understanding the underlying mechanisms and implementing lifestyle modifications and medical

interventions, individuals with acid reflux and GERD can find relief and promote a healthier digestive system.
•	Understanding Acid Reflux and GERD:
We will begin by defining acid reflux and GERD and explaining the difference between the two conditions. We will explore the anatomical structures involved, including the lower esophageal sphincter (LES) and the role of stomach acid in the reflux process.
•	Causes and Triggers of Acid Reflux and GERD:
We will discuss the common causes and triggers of acid reflux and GERD. Factors such as certain foods, obesity, smoking, pregnancy, and hiatal hernias can contribute to the development or exacerbation of these conditions.
•	Symptoms and Complications:
We will delve into the symptoms of acid reflux and GERD, including heartburn, regurgitation, chest pain, difficulty swallowing, and chronic cough. We will also discuss potential complications, such as esophagitis, Barrett's esophagus, and respiratory issues.
•	Lifestyle Modifications for Managing Acid Reflux and GERD:
We will explore various lifestyle modifications that can help alleviate symptoms and reduce the frequency of reflux episodes. This will include dietary changes, such as avoiding trigger foods, eating smaller meals, maintaining a healthy weight, and practicing proper mealtime habits.
•	Dietary Approaches for Acid Reflux and GERD:
We will discuss specific dietary approaches that can help soothe the flames of acid reflux and GERD. This will include recommendations for reducing the intake of acidic and spicy foods, caffeine, alcohol, and fatty foods. We will also explore the benefits of incorporating more fiber-rich foods and alkaline-forming foods into the diet.
•	Managing Nighttime Acid Reflux:
Nighttime acid reflux can disrupt sleep and worsen symptoms. We will provide strategies for managing nighttime reflux, such as adjusting sleeping positions, using

elevation devices, and implementing proper timing of meals and snacks.
•   Medications for Acid Reflux and GERD:
We will discuss the different types of medications used in the management of acid reflux and GERD. This will include antacids, H2 blockers, proton pump inhibitors (PPIs), and prokinetics. We will explore their mechanisms of action, potential side effects, and appropriate usage.
•   Surgical Interventions for Acid Reflux and GERD:
In some cases, surgical intervention may be necessary for individuals with severe or persistent symptoms. We will discuss surgical options such as fundoplication and LINX procedure and their role in managing acid reflux and GERD.
•   Alternative Therapies and Natural Remedies:
We will explore alternative therapies and natural remedies that may help soothe the symptoms of acid reflux and GERD. This will include approaches such as herbal supplements, acupuncture, relaxation techniques, and homeopathic remedies. We will discuss the available evidence and their potential benefits in managing these conditions.

Acid reflux and GERD can significantly impact daily life, but with proper management strategies, individuals can find relief and improve their digestive health. By implementing lifestyle modifications, dietary changes, and utilizing appropriate medications or surgical interventions when necessary, individuals with acid reflux and GERD can soothe the flames, reduce symptoms, and promote a healthier digestive system. It is essential to work closely with healthcare professionals to develop a personalized management plan that addresses individual needs and preferences.

6.4 Celiac Disease: Navigating a Gluten-Free Lifestyle

Celiac disease is an autoimmune disorder triggered by the consumption of gluten, a protein found in wheat, barley, and rye. In this chapter, "Celiac Disease: Navigating a Gluten-Free Lifestyle," we will explore the intricacies of celiac disease, including its causes, symptoms, diagnosis, and effective strategies for managing the condition through a gluten-free lifestyle. By understanding the impact of celiac disease on the body and implementing dietary changes, individuals with celiac disease can lead healthy, symptom-free lives.

• Understanding Celiac Disease:

We will begin by providing a comprehensive overview of celiac disease, including its definition, prevalence, and the immune response triggered by gluten consumption. We will also discuss the genetic and environmental factors that contribute to the development of celiac disease.

• Symptoms and Complications:

We will explore the wide range of symptoms associated with celiac disease, which can vary from gastrointestinal issues such as diarrhea, abdominal pain, and bloating to non-gastrointestinal symptoms like fatigue, anemia, skin rashes, and neurological manifestations. We will also discuss potential complications, such as malabsorption, nutrient deficiencies, osteoporosis, and increased risk of certain autoimmune disorders.

• Diagnostic Process:

We will delve into the diagnostic process for celiac disease, including the importance of recognizing symptoms, undergoing serological tests, and confirming the diagnosis through intestinal biopsy. We will also discuss the significance of genetic testing and the role of healthcare professionals in guiding the diagnostic journey.

• Gluten-Free Diet Essentials:

We will provide a comprehensive guide to adopting and maintaining a gluten-free lifestyle. This will include an in-depth understanding of gluten-containing foods, hidden sources of gluten, and label reading. We will also discuss the importance of cross-contamination prevention, safe food preparation, and strategies for dining out.

• Gluten-Free Food Substitutions and Alternatives:

To ensure a well-rounded and enjoyable gluten-free diet, we will explore a variety of gluten-free substitutes and alternatives for common gluten-containing foods. This will include grains, flours, bread, pasta, baked goods, and condiments. We will also discuss the nutritional value and taste profiles of different gluten-free options.

•	Meeting Nutritional Needs:
We will address the potential challenges individuals with celiac disease may face in meeting their nutritional needs. This will include recommendations for obtaining essential nutrients such as fiber, vitamins, and minerals through gluten-free food choices, as well as the potential need for dietary supplementation.

•	Managing Social and Emotional Aspects:
Living with celiac disease can present unique social and emotional challenges. We will discuss strategies for navigating social situations, dining out, and traveling while adhering to a gluten-free lifestyle. Additionally, we will address the emotional impact of celiac disease and provide guidance on finding support networks and coping with the psychological aspects of the condition.

•	Long-Term Health and Monitoring:
We will emphasize the importance of long-term health management for individuals with celiac disease. This will include regular follow-up visits, monitoring nutritional status, assessing for potential complications, and understanding the potential for associated conditions such as dermatitis herpetiformis and gluten ataxia.

•	Research and Future Developments:
We will discuss current research trends and potential future developments in celiac disease management. This will include advancements in diagnostic methods, treatment options, and the exploration of non-dietary therapies.

Celiac disease necessitates a lifelong commitment to a gluten-free lifestyle. By understanding the intricacies of the condition, adhering to a strict gluten-free diet, seeking appropriate medical care, and addressing the social and emotional aspects, individuals with celiac disease can navigate their way to a healthy and fulfilling life. With ongoing research and support, the future holds promise for improved diagnostics, treatment options, and increased awareness of celiac disease and its management.

6.5 Gut Health and Food Allergies

Food allergies are a growing concern worldwide, affecting millions of people. In this chapter, "Gut Health and Food Allergies," we will explore the intricate relationship between the gut and food allergies. We will delve into the mechanisms of food allergies, the role of the gut in immune responses, and strategies for managing food allergies through gut health optimization. By understanding the connection between the gut and food allergies, individuals can take proactive steps to promote a healthier gut and reduce the risk and impact of food allergies.
- Understanding Food Allergies:
We will provide a comprehensive overview of food allergies, including the definition, common allergenic foods, prevalence, and symptoms associated with allergic reactions. We will also discuss the difference between food allergies and other adverse reactions to food, such as food intolerances.
- The Gut-Immune System Connection:
We will explore the intricate relationship between the gut and the immune system. This will include an overview of the gut-associated lymphoid tissue (GALT), the role of gut microbiota in immune regulation, and the development of oral tolerance. We will also discuss how disturbances in gut health can contribute to the development or exacerbation of food allergies.
- Gut Health and Food Allergy Development:
We will delve into the factors that influence the development of food allergies, with a particular focus on the role of gut health. This will include the impact of early-life gut microbial

colonization, the hygiene hypothesis, and the potential link between gut permeability (leaky gut) and food allergies.
- Strategies for Gut Health Optimization:
We will discuss various strategies to optimize gut health and promote a balanced immune response to reduce the risk and severity of food allergies. This will include dietary interventions, such as the inclusion of prebiotic and probiotic-rich foods, as well as the importance of fiber, antioxidants, and omega-3 fatty acids. We will also explore lifestyle factors, including stress management, regular exercise, and adequate sleep, that contribute to a healthy gut environment.
- Gut Health and the Prevention of Food Allergies:
We will discuss the potential role of gut health in the prevention of food allergies, particularly in high-risk individuals such as infants and children. This will include breastfeeding, introduction of complementary foods, and the timing of allergenic food introduction. We will also discuss the evolving field of oral immunotherapy and its potential for desensitization and prevention of food allergies.
- Managing Food Allergies through Gut Health Optimization:
For individuals already diagnosed with food allergies, we will explore how optimizing gut health can complement existing management strategies. This will include dietary modifications, such as avoiding trigger foods, supporting gut barrier function, and reducing inflammation. We will also discuss potential therapeutic interventions, including targeted probiotic and prebiotic supplementation, and their role in managing food allergies.
- Gut Health and the Gut-Brain Axis in Food Allergies:
We will touch upon the gut-brain axis and its influence on food allergies. This will include the potential impact of stress, anxiety, and psychological factors on the severity of allergic reactions. We will also discuss strategies for managing stress and promoting emotional well-being to support overall gut health and food allergy management.

- Working with Healthcare Professionals: We will emphasize the importance of working with healthcare professionals in the diagnosis, management, and treatment of food allergies. This will include allergists, gastroenterologists, dietitians, and other specialists who can provide guidance and personalized recommendations for optimizing gut health and managing food allergies.

Understanding the complex relationship between the gut and food allergies is crucial for individuals with allergies and healthcare professionals. By prioritizing gut health through dietary and lifestyle interventions, individuals can support a balanced immune response, reduce the risk of food allergies, and better manage existing allergies. Ongoing research in this field holds promise for further advancements in the prevention and management of food allergies through gut health optimization.

Chapter 7

<u>Gut Health Across the Lifespan</u>

7.1 Gut Health during Pregnancy and Postpartum

The journey of pregnancy and the postpartum period bring significant changes to a woman's body, including the gut microbiome. In this chapter, "Gut Health during Pregnancy and Postpartum," we will explore the impact of pregnancy and childbirth on gut health. We will discuss the dynamic interplay between the gut microbiota, hormonal changes, immune function, and maternal health during this transformative period. By understanding the unique considerations and implementing strategies for promoting gut health, women can support their own well-being and lay a foundation for their baby's health.

- Gut Health and Pregnancy:

We will provide an overview of the changes that occur in the gut microbiome during pregnancy. This will include the impact of hormonal fluctuations, immune modulation, and dietary changes on the composition and diversity of the gut microbiota. We will also discuss the potential implications of these changes for maternal health and pregnancy outcomes.

- Gut Health and Maternal Well-being:

We will explore the bidirectional relationship between gut health and maternal well-being during pregnancy and postpartum. This will include the potential impact of gut dysbiosis on mood disorders, such as prenatal and postpartum depression and anxiety. We will also discuss strategies for promoting a healthy gut microbiome to support maternal mental health.

- Nutrition for Gut Health during Pregnancy:

We will discuss the importance of nutrition in supporting gut health during pregnancy. This will include dietary recommendations for promoting a diverse and balanced gut microbiota, including the consumption of prebiotic and probiotic-rich foods, fiber, and essential nutrients. We will also address common dietary challenges and considerations during pregnancy.

- The Gut-Maternal-Fetal Axis:

We will explore the emerging concept of the gut-maternal-fetal axis and its role in influencing the development and health of the baby. This will include discussions on maternal transmission of microbiota, the potential impact of the maternal gut microbiome on the baby's immune system, and the importance of maternal gut health in shaping the infant's microbiome.

- Gut Health during Labor and Delivery:

We will discuss the impact of labor and delivery on gut health, both for the mother and the baby. This will include the potential transmission of beneficial bacteria during vaginal birth and the impact of cesarean section on the establishment of the baby's gut microbiota. We will also explore strategies to promote a healthy gut microbiome in newborns delivered via cesarean section.

- Gut Health in the Postpartum Period:

We will focus on the unique considerations for gut health during the postpartum period. This will include discussions on hormonal changes, breastfeeding, and the potential impact of stress and sleep deprivation on gut health. We will also provide practical tips for supporting gut health in the postpartum period, including dietary recommendations, probiotic supplementation, and self-care practices.

- Optimizing Gut Health for Maternal-Infant Health:

We will emphasize the importance of optimizing gut health for both maternal and infant well-being. This will include discussions on the potential long-term health implications of the maternal gut microbiome for the baby, strategies for breastfeeding support to promote a healthy infant gut microbiome, and the role of probiotics in maternal and infant gut health.

- Gut Health Considerations for Assisted Reproductive Technologies:

We will touch upon the unique considerations for gut health in individuals undergoing assisted reproductive technologies (ART). This will include the potential impact of ART procedures, medications, and stress on the gut microbiome. We will also discuss strategies to support gut health in individuals undergoing fertility treatments.

During pregnancy and the postpartum period, gut health plays a crucial role in supporting maternal well-being and laying the foundation for the baby's health. By implementing strategies to promote a healthy gut microbiome, such as proper nutrition, probiotic supplementation, and self-care practices, women can optimize their gut health and contribute to positive outcomes for themselves and their babies. Ongoing research in this field will continue to shed light on the intricate connections between gut health, pregnancy, and early-life development.

7.2 Nurturing a Healthy Gut in Infants and Children

The early years of life are critical for the development and establishment of a healthy gut microbiome, which plays a crucial role in overall health and well-being. In this chapter, "Nurturing a Healthy Gut in Infants and Children," we will explore the factors that influence gut health during this formative stage of life. We will discuss the importance of breastfeeding, introduction of solid foods, dietary choices, and environmental factors in shaping a diverse and resilient gut microbiome. By understanding the key principles and strategies for nurturing a healthy gut in infants and children, parents and caregivers can support optimal growth, development, and long-term health.

- The Role of the Gut Microbiome in Early Life:

We will provide an overview of the importance of the gut microbiome in early life and its impact on various aspects of health, including immune system development, metabolism, and brain development. We will also discuss the concept of the "microbiome-gut-brain axis" and how early-life gut health influences cognitive and emotional well-being.

- Breastfeeding and Gut Health:

We will discuss the unique benefits of breastfeeding for gut health in infants. This will include the composition of breast milk, which provides essential nutrients, prebiotics, and immune factors that support the growth of beneficial gut bacteria. We will also address common challenges in breastfeeding and provide guidance for promoting successful breastfeeding practices.

- Introduction of Solid Foods:

We will explore the transition from exclusive breastfeeding or formula feeding to the introduction of solid foods. This will include discussions on the timing, diversity, and nutrient density of complementary foods to promote a healthy gut microbiome. We will also address common concerns, such as food allergies and intolerances, and provide guidance on introducing allergenic foods.

- The Importance of Fiber for Gut Health:

We will emphasize the role of dietary fiber in supporting a healthy gut microbiome in infants and children. This will include discussions on age-appropriate sources of fiber, such as fruits, vegetables, whole grains, and legumes. We will also provide practical tips for increasing fiber intake in children's diets.

- Probiotics and Gut Health in Infants and Children:

We will explore the role of probiotics in supporting gut health in infants and children. This will include discussions on specific strains, their potential benefits, and safety considerations. We will also address the use of probiotics in managing common childhood conditions, such as colic, diarrhea, and antibiotic-associated gastrointestinal disturbances.

- Environmental Factors and Gut Health:

We will discuss the impact of environmental factors on gut health in infants and children. This will include the potential influence of antibiotics, exposure to chemicals and toxins, and the role of a hygienic versus a microbial-rich environment in the development of a robust and diverse gut microbiome. We will also provide practical tips for creating a healthy and supportive environment for gut health.

•   Supporting Gut Health in Picky Eaters:
We will address the challenges of feeding picky eaters and provide strategies for promoting a diverse and nutritious diet to support gut health. This will include discussions on fostering a positive food environment, involving children in meal planning and preparation, and addressing sensory and texture preferences.

•   Gut Health and the Developing Immune System:
We will explore the interplay between gut health and the developing immune system in infants and children. This will include discussions on the role of the gut microbiome in immune system maturation, the prevention of allergies and autoimmune disorders, and strategies for supporting a balanced immune response through gut health optimization.

Nurturing a healthy gut in infants and children is crucial for their overall growth, development, and long-term health. By understanding the key principles of breastfeeding, introducing appropriate solid foods, emphasizing fiber-rich diets, considering probiotic supplementation, and addressing environmental factors, parents and caregivers can lay a strong foundation for optimal gut health in their children. Ongoing research in this field will continue to provide valuable insights into the intricate relationship between gut health and childhood well-being.

7.3 Gut Health in Adolescents: Navigating Hormonal Changes

Adolescence is a period of significant physiological and psychological changes, including the onset of puberty and hormonal fluctuations. These changes can have a profound impact on gut health and overall well-being. In this chapter, "Gut Health in Adolescents: Navigating Hormonal Changes," we will explore the unique considerations for gut health during this transitional stage of life. We will discuss the effects of hormonal changes on the gut microbiome, the gut-brain axis, and immune function. We will also provide strategies to support gut health and promote a healthy balance during adolescence.

- Puberty and Gut Microbiome:
We will explore the influence of puberty on the gut microbiome. This will include discussions on the hormonal changes that occur during this stage and how they can affect the composition and diversity of gut bacteria. We will also address the potential impact of these changes on digestive function, metabolism, and overall gut health.
- Gut Health and Hormonal Balance:
We will discuss the bidirectional relationship between gut health and hormonal balance during adolescence. This will include the role of the gut microbiome in metabolizing hormones, such as estrogen and testosterone, and the impact of hormonal imbalances on gut health. We will also explore strategies to support hormonal balance through gut health optimization.
- Gut-Brain Axis and Emotional Well-being:
We will explore the connection between the gut and the brain during adolescence, emphasizing the impact of hormonal changes on emotional well-being. This will include discussions on the role of the gut microbiome in neurotransmitter production, stress response, and mood regulation. We will provide strategies to support a healthy gut-brain axis and promote emotional balance during this critical stage.
- Nutrition for Gut Health in Adolescents:
We will discuss the importance of nutrition in supporting gut health during adolescence. This will include discussions on nutrient-dense foods, fiber intake, and the consumption of prebiotic and probiotic-rich foods. We will also address

common dietary challenges during this stage, such as restrictive eating patterns and poor food choices, and provide guidance for promoting a balanced and gut-friendly diet.

- Gut Health and Immune Function:
We will explore the interplay between gut health and immune function during adolescence. This will include discussions on the gut microbiome's role in immune system development, allergic responses, and inflammatory conditions. We will also discuss strategies to support a healthy immune system through gut health optimization.

- Gut Health and Digestive Disorders in Adolescents:
We will address the prevalence and management of digestive disorders, such as irritable bowel syndrome (IBS) and inflammatory bowel disease (IBD), in adolescents. This will include discussions on the potential impact of hormonal changes on the development and management of these conditions. We will provide strategies for promoting gut health and managing digestive disorders during this stage of life.

- Lifestyle Factors for Gut Health:
We will emphasize the importance of lifestyle factors in supporting gut health during adolescence. This will include discussions on physical activity, stress management, sleep hygiene, and environmental factors. We will provide practical tips for incorporating these lifestyle factors into daily routines to promote a healthy gut and overall well-being.

- Promoting Gut Health in School Settings:
We will discuss the role of schools in promoting gut health among adolescents. This will include discussions on nutrition education, access to gut-friendly foods in school cafeterias, and the importance of creating supportive environments for gut health. We will also address the challenges and opportunities for promoting gut health within the school setting.

Navigating the hormonal changes of adolescence can be challenging, but by understanding the impact of these changes on gut health and implementing strategies to support a healthy gut microbiome, adolescents can optimize their overall well-being. By emphasizing nutrition, addressing hormonal balance, supporting the gut-brain axis, and considering lifestyle factors, adolescents can navigate this transitional period with improved gut health and resilience. Ongoing research in this field will continue to shed light on the unique considerations and opportunities for promoting gut health during adolescence.

7.4: Gut Health for Adults: Maintaining Balance in Busy Lives

In today's fast-paced and demanding world, adults often face numerous challenges when it comes to maintaining a healthy gut. Stress, poor dietary choices, sedentary lifestyles, and environmental factors can all take a toll on gut health. In this chapter, "Gut Health for Adults: Maintaining Balance in Busy Lives," we will explore the key considerations and strategies for promoting gut health in adulthood. We will discuss the impact of lifestyle factors, stress management, nutrition, and the gut-brain axis on maintaining a balanced gut microbiome. By incorporating practical approaches, adults can prioritize their gut health and enhance their overall well-being.
•   The Gut Microbiome in Adulthood:
We will provide an overview of the gut microbiome in adulthood, discussing its composition, diversity, and role in overall health. We will explore the factors that can influence the gut microbiome during this stage of life, such as diet, medications, and environmental exposures. Understanding the unique characteristics of the adult gut microbiome will lay the foundation for implementing effective gut health strategies.
•   Nutrition for Gut Health:

We will delve into the role of nutrition in supporting gut health in adults. This will include discussions on the importance of a balanced diet rich in fiber, prebiotics, and probiotics. We will explore the impact of dietary choices on gut microbial diversity, inflammation, and chronic diseases. Practical tips for incorporating gut-friendly foods into busy lifestyles will be provided.

- Stress Management and Gut Health:

We will examine the relationship between stress and gut health in adults. Chronic stress can disrupt the delicate balance of the gut microbiome and contribute to digestive issues. We will discuss the mechanisms through which stress affects the gut, including the gut-brain axis and the release of stress hormones. Strategies for stress reduction and resilience-building techniques will be explored.

- Gut Health and Digestive Disorders:

We will address common digestive disorders that affect adults, such as irritable bowel syndrome (IBS), acid reflux, and inflammatory bowel disease (IBD). Understanding the symptoms, triggers, and management approaches for these conditions will empower individuals to take proactive steps in maintaining gut health. We will discuss the importance of seeking professional guidance and individualized approaches to manage specific digestive disorders.

- Lifestyle Factors for Gut Health:

We will emphasize the significance of lifestyle factors in supporting gut health for adults. This will include discussions on physical activity, sleep hygiene, smoking cessation, and alcohol moderation. We will explore the impact of these lifestyle choices on gut motility, inflammation, and gut microbial balance. Practical suggestions for incorporating these factors into busy lives will be provided.

- Gut Health and Immune Function:

We will examine the interplay between gut health and immune function in adults. A healthy gut microbiome plays a vital role in maintaining a balanced immune response and defending against pathogens. We will discuss the impact of gut dysbiosis on immune-related disorders and explore strategies to support immune health through gut health optimization.

•   Gut Health and Mental Well-being:
We will explore the connection between gut health and mental well-being in adults. The gut-brain axis influences mood, cognition, and emotional balance. We will discuss the impact of the gut microbiome on neurotransmitter production, inflammation, and stress response. Strategies for nurturing a healthy gut-brain axis and promoting mental well-being will be discussed.

•   Environmental Factors and Gut Health:
We will address the impact of environmental factors on gut health in adults. This will include discussions on the role of pollutants, medications, and food additives in gut dysbiosis. We will explore strategies for minimizing exposure to harmful substances and creating a gut-friendly living environment.

Maintaining a healthy gut in adulthood is a multifaceted endeavor that requires attention to nutrition, stress management, lifestyle factors, and environmental influences. By prioritizing gut health and implementing practical strategies, adults can optimize their overall well-being and prevent the onset of gut-related disorders. Ongoing research in this field will continue to provide insights into the intricate connections between gut health and adult health.

7.5 Aging Gracefully: Gut Health for Seniors

As we age, maintaining good gut health becomes increasingly important for overall well-being and quality of life. The aging process can bring changes to the gut microbiome, digestion, and immune function, which may impact gut health. In this chapter, "Aging Gracefully: Gut Health for Seniors," we will explore the unique considerations and strategies for promoting optimal gut health in the senior population. We will discuss the impact of aging on the gut microbiome, nutrient absorption, digestive function, and immune response. By implementing targeted approaches, seniors can support their gut health and enhance their overall health and vitality.

•   Age-Related Changes in the Gut Microbiome: We will explore the impact of aging on the composition and diversity of the gut microbiome. Age-related factors, such as diet, medications, and immune function, can affect the balance of gut bacteria. We will discuss the potential consequences of these changes and explore strategies to promote a healthy and resilient gut microbiome in seniors.

•   Nutrient Absorption and Gut Health: We will delve into the challenges and considerations related to nutrient absorption in seniors. Age-related changes in digestive enzymes, stomach acid production, and gut motility can affect the absorption of essential nutrients. We will discuss the importance of optimizing nutrient intake and explore strategies to enhance nutrient absorption for better gut health.

•   Digestive Health and Senior-specific Issues: We will address common digestive issues that affect seniors, such as constipation, acid reflux, and diverticulosis. We will discuss the potential causes and management approaches for these conditions, with an emphasis on maintaining gut health. Practical tips for promoting regularity, reducing discomfort, and optimizing digestion in seniors will be provided.

•   Immune Function and Gut Health in Seniors: We will examine the impact of aging on immune function and its relationship with gut health. The gut plays a crucial role in immune response, and age-related changes can impact immune function. We will discuss strategies to support a robust immune system through gut health optimization, including dietary choices and lifestyle factors.

•   Nutrition and Hydration for Senior Gut Health:

We will explore the role of nutrition and hydration in promoting gut health in seniors. Age-related changes in appetite, taste, and oral health can affect dietary choices and nutrient intake. We will discuss the importance of a well-balanced diet, adequate fiber intake, and hydration for maintaining a healthy gut and preventing digestive issues.

- Managing Medications and Gut Health:

We will address the impact of medications on gut health in seniors. Polypharmacy, or the use of multiple medications, is common among seniors and can have implications for gut health. We will discuss strategies to minimize medication-related disruptions to gut health, such as discussing potential side effects with healthcare providers and considering probiotic supplementation.

- Maintaining Physical Activity and Gut Health:

We will emphasize the significance of physical activity in supporting gut health in seniors. Regular exercise can enhance gut motility, reduce inflammation, and promote overall well-being. We will discuss the benefits of different types of exercise for gut health and provide practical suggestions for incorporating physical activity into a senior's daily routine.

- Mental and Emotional Well-being in Senior Gut Health:

We will explore the connection between gut health and mental and emotional well-being in seniors. Age-related factors, such as loneliness, stress, and cognitive decline, can impact gut health and vice versa. We will discuss strategies for nurturing a healthy gut-brain axis, promoting emotional well-being, and supporting mental clarity in seniors.

Maintaining a healthy gut is essential for seniors to age gracefully and enjoy a high quality of life. By understanding the unique considerations and implementing targeted strategies for gut health, seniors can optimize digestion, nutrient absorption, immune function, and overall well-being. Ongoing research in this field will continue to provide insights into the specific needs and opportunities for promoting gut health in the senior population.

Chapter 8

<u>Gut Health and Weight Management</u>

8.1 Gut Microbiome and Metabolism

Maintaining a healthy weight is a goal for many individuals, and understanding the role of gut health in weight management is crucial. The gut microbiome, with its intricate connections to metabolism, plays a significant role in regulating body weight. In this chapter, "Gut Health and Weight Management," we will explore the relationship between the gut microbiome and metabolism, the impact of gut dysbiosis on weight gain, and strategies for optimizing gut health to support healthy weight management.

•   The Gut Microbiome and Energy Balance: We will provide an overview of the gut microbiome's role in energy balance and metabolism. The gut microbiome influences the extraction and storage of energy from food, as well as the regulation of appetite and satiety signals. We will explore the mechanisms through which the gut microbiome influences weight regulation and metabolism.

•   Gut Dysbiosis and Weight Gain: We will discuss the impact of gut dysbiosis, an imbalance in the gut microbial composition, on weight gain and obesity. Disruptions in the gut microbiome can lead to increased calorie extraction from food, inflammation, and metabolic dysfunction, contributing to weight gain. We will explore the factors that can contribute to gut dysbiosis and the implications for weight management.

•   Gut Health Strategies for Weight Loss:

We will discuss strategies for optimizing gut health to support weight loss efforts. This will include discussions on dietary interventions, such as incorporating fiber-rich foods, prebiotics, and probiotics, to promote a diverse and healthy gut microbiome. We will explore the potential benefits of specific dietary patterns, such as the Mediterranean diet or a plant-based diet, for weight management and gut health.

•	Gut Health and Appetite Regulation:
We will examine the connection between gut health and appetite regulation. The gut microbiome plays a role in producing signaling molecules that regulate hunger and fullness. We will discuss how gut dysbiosis can disrupt this signaling and contribute to overeating or poor appetite control. Strategies for improving appetite regulation through gut health optimization will be explored.

•	Exercise, Gut Health, and Weight Management:
We will explore the relationship between exercise, gut health, and weight management. Regular physical activity can influence the gut microbiome, improve gut motility, and support metabolic health. We will discuss the potential benefits of exercise for gut health and weight management, as well as practical suggestions for incorporating exercise into a weight loss plan.

•	Gut Health and Emotional Eating:
We will address the impact of emotional eating on gut health and weight management. Stress, emotional states, and disordered eating patterns can disrupt the gut microbiome and contribute to weight gain. We will explore strategies for managing emotional eating, stress reduction, and nurturing a healthy gut-brain axis to support weight management goals.

•	Long-Term Weight Maintenance and Gut Health:
We will discuss the importance of maintaining gut health for sustainable weight management. Long-term weight maintenance requires ongoing support for a healthy gut microbiome. We will explore strategies for sustaining gut health, including lifestyle factors, stress management, and maintaining a balanced diet.

- Gut Health and Bariatric Surgery:
We will examine the impact of bariatric surgery on gut health and weight management. Bariatric procedures can significantly alter the gut microbiome and metabolic pathways, leading to weight loss. We will discuss the potential effects of bariatric surgery on gut health, nutrient absorption, and long-term weight management.

Optimizing gut health is crucial for effective weight management. By understanding the connections between the gut microbiome, metabolism, appetite regulation, and emotional well-being, individuals can implement targeted strategies to support healthy weight loss and long-term weight maintenance. Ongoing research in this field will continue to provide insights into the potential of gut health interventions for weight management.

8.2 Gut Health Strategies for Healthy Weight Loss

Weight loss is a common goal for many individuals, and optimizing gut health can play a crucial role in achieving sustainable and healthy weight loss. In this chapter, "Gut Health Strategies for Healthy Weight Loss," we will explore various strategies and interventions that promote a healthy gut microbiome, enhance metabolism, and support successful weight loss. By understanding the connections between gut health and weight management, individuals can implement evidence-based strategies to achieve their weight loss goals.

- Assessing Gut Health for Weight Loss:
We will discuss the importance of assessing gut health before embarking on a weight loss journey. Understanding the current state of the gut microbiome and identifying any imbalances or dysbiosis can help tailor interventions for optimal results. We will explore different methods of assessing gut health, including microbiome testing and symptom assessment.

- Dietary Approaches for Gut Health and Weight Loss:

We will explore various dietary approaches that promote both gut health and weight loss. This will include discussions on the benefits of fiber-rich foods, whole grains, fruits, and vegetables for nourishing the gut microbiome. We will also explore the potential benefits of specific dietary patterns, such as a low-carbohydrate diet, a Mediterranean-style diet, or intermittent fasting, for weight loss and gut health.

- Probiotics and Weight Loss:

We will delve into the role of probiotics in supporting healthy weight loss. Probiotics are beneficial bacteria that can help restore and maintain a healthy gut microbiome. We will discuss specific strains of probiotics that have shown promise in supporting weight loss efforts and explore their mechanisms of action.

- Prebiotics and Weight Loss:

We will explore the role of prebiotics in promoting gut health and weight loss. Prebiotics are non-digestible fibers that serve as food for beneficial gut bacteria. We will discuss how prebiotics can stimulate the growth of beneficial bacteria, improve gut barrier function, and support weight loss efforts. Dietary sources of prebiotics and their inclusion in a weight loss diet will be explored.

- Gut Health and Metabolism:

We will examine the connections between gut health and metabolism in the context of weight loss. A healthy gut microbiome plays a role in regulating metabolic pathways and energy utilization. We will discuss the impact of gut dysbiosis on metabolism and explore strategies for optimizing gut health to enhance metabolic function and support weight loss.

- Lifestyle Factors for Gut Health and Weight Loss:

We will discuss the importance of lifestyle factors in supporting both gut health and weight loss. Adequate sleep, stress management, regular physical activity, and healthy habits all contribute to a healthy gut microbiome and

facilitate weight loss. We will explore practical strategies for incorporating these lifestyle factors into a weight loss plan.
•	Mindful Eating for Gut Health and Weight Loss: We will emphasize the importance of mindful eating in promoting both gut health and weight loss. Mindful eating involves paying attention to hunger cues, eating slowly, and savoring each bite. We will discuss how mindful eating can enhance digestion, improve nutrient absorption, and support weight loss efforts. Practical tips for practicing mindful eating will be provided.

•	Monitoring Progress and Adjusting Interventions: We will explore the importance of monitoring progress and adjusting interventions throughout the weight loss journey. Regular assessments of gut health, body composition, and weight can help determine the effectiveness of the implemented strategies. We will discuss how to make informed decisions about adjusting dietary choices, supplementation, and lifestyle factors to optimize gut health and maximize weight loss outcomes.
Conclusion:
Optimizing gut health is a key component of achieving healthy and sustainable weight loss. By implementing targeted strategies that nourish the gut microbiome, enhance metabolism, and support overall well-being, individuals can improve their chances of successful weight loss. The integration of dietary modifications, probiotics, prebiotics, lifestyle changes, and mindful eating practices can create a synergistic effect to support gut health and facilitate weight loss. Ongoing research in this field will continue to provide insights and innovations for promoting healthy weight loss through gut health optimization.

Chapter 8.3: Gut Health and Weight Gain: Identifying Contributing Factors

Weight gain is a complex issue influenced by various factors, including diet, lifestyle, genetics, and gut health. In this chapter, "Gut Health and Weight Gain: Identifying Contributing Factors," we will explore the role of gut health in weight gain and discuss the underlying mechanisms that contribute to excessive weight gain. By understanding these factors, individuals can take proactive steps to address gut health and mitigate the risk of weight gain.

- Gut Microbiome and Weight Gain:
We will discuss the relationship between the gut microbiome and weight gain. The composition of the gut microbiome can influence energy extraction from food, metabolic pathways, and the regulation of appetite. We will explore how imbalances or dysbiosis in the gut microbiome can lead to increased calorie absorption, inflammation, and metabolic dysfunction, all of which contribute to weight gain.

- Gut Dysbiosis and Weight Gain:
We will examine the impact of gut dysbiosis on weight gain. Disruptions in the gut microbiome, such as an overgrowth of harmful bacteria or a reduction in beneficial bacteria, can affect energy balance, nutrient absorption, and inflammation, leading to weight gain. We will discuss the factors that contribute to gut dysbiosis, including poor diet, stress, medication use, and environmental influences.

- Inflammation and Weight Gain:
We will explore the connection between inflammation and weight gain. Chronic low-grade inflammation in the body, often driven by gut dysbiosis, can disrupt metabolic pathways and contribute to weight gain. We will discuss the role of inflammatory markers, such as C-reactive protein (CRP), in assessing inflammation levels and their association with weight gain.

- Gut Permeability and Weight Gain:

We will delve into the concept of gut permeability, also known as "leaky gut," and its association with weight gain. Increased gut permeability allows harmful substances to enter the bloodstream, triggering an immune response and promoting inflammation. We will discuss how gut permeability can contribute to weight gain and strategies for improving gut barrier function.

- Gut Health and Hormonal Imbalance: We will examine the impact of gut health on hormonal balance and weight gain. The gut microbiome plays a role in regulating hormones related to appetite, satiety, and metabolism, such as leptin and ghrelin. We will discuss how gut dysbiosis can disrupt these hormonal signals, leading to increased food cravings, overeating, and weight gain.
- Medications and Weight Gain: We will explore the impact of certain medications on gut health and weight gain. Some medications, such as antibiotics, proton pump inhibitors (PPIs), and antidepressants, can disrupt the gut microbiome and contribute to weight gain. We will discuss strategies for mitigating the effects of these medications on gut health and weight management.
- Stress, Gut Health, and Weight Gain: We will discuss the intricate relationship between stress, gut health, and weight gain. Chronic stress can disrupt the gut microbiome, impair digestion, and promote weight gain. We will explore stress management techniques and strategies for nurturing a healthy gut-brain axis to support weight management goals.
- Genetic Factors and Gut Health: We will examine the influence of genetic factors on gut health and weight gain. Genetic variations can impact an individual's susceptibility to gut dysbiosis, inflammation, and metabolic dysfunction, leading to weight gain. We will discuss the potential role of genetic testing in identifying genetic predispositions and tailoring interventions for optimal weight management.

Understanding the connections between gut health and weight gain is essential for addressing the underlying factors contributing to excessive weight gain. By considering the impact of the gut microbiome, inflammation, gut permeability, hormonal balance, medications, stress, and genetic factors, individuals can take proactive steps to support gut health and mitigate the risk of weight gain. Implementing strategies to optimize gut health, such as dietary modifications, stress management, and targeted supplementation, can contribute to maintaining a healthy weight and overall well-being.

8.4 Emotional Eating and Gut Health

Emotional eating refers to the tendency to eat in response to emotions rather than physical hunger. It is a common behavior that can have a significant impact on overall health and weight management. In this chapter, "Emotional Eating and Gut Health," we will explore the complex relationship between emotional eating, gut health, and its implications for well-being. Understanding this connection is crucial for developing strategies to address emotional eating and promote a healthy gut.

- Emotional Eating: Understanding the Behavior: We will delve into the concept of emotional eating, exploring the reasons behind this behavior. Emotional eating often involves consuming high-calorie, comfort foods as a means to cope with stress, sadness, boredom, or other emotions. We will discuss the psychological and physiological factors that contribute to emotional eating and its potential impact on gut health.
- Gut-Brain Axis and Emotional Eating: We will explore the bidirectional communication between the gut and the brain, known as the gut-brain axis, and its role in emotional eating. The gut-brain axis involves complex interactions between the gut microbiota, the enteric nervous system, and the central nervous system. We will discuss how imbalances in the gut microbiome and

disruptions in the gut-brain communication can influence emotional eating behaviors.
•	Gut Microbiome and Mood:
We will examine the impact of the gut microbiome on mood and emotions. Emerging research suggests that the gut microbiota can produce neurotransmitters and other signaling molecules that influence brain function and mood. We will discuss how imbalances in the gut microbiome, such as dysbiosis or reduced microbial diversity, can affect emotional well-being and potentially contribute to emotional eating.
•	Stress, Gut Health, and Emotional Eating:
We will explore the intricate relationship between stress, gut health, and emotional eating. Chronic stress can disrupt the gut microbiome, compromise gut barrier function, and promote inflammation, all of which can influence emotional eating behaviors. We will discuss stress management techniques and strategies for nurturing a healthy gut-brain axis to address emotional eating patterns.
•	Food Cravings and Gut Health:
We will discuss the relationship between food cravings, gut health, and emotional eating. Certain gut microbes and their metabolites can influence food preferences and cravings, potentially driving emotional eating behaviors. We will explore strategies for managing food cravings and supporting a balanced gut microbiome to mitigate the impact of cravings on emotional eating.
•	Mindful Eating and Gut Health:
We will explore the practice of mindful eating as a tool for addressing emotional eating and promoting gut health. Mindful eating involves cultivating awareness and non-judgmental attention to the eating experience. We will discuss how mindful eating practices can help individuals develop a healthier relationship with food, enhance digestion, and promote a balanced gut-brain connection.
•	Gut-Healthy Nutrition for Emotional Well-being:
We will examine the role of nutrition in supporting emotional well-being and addressing emotional eating. Certain

nutrients, such as omega-3 fatty acids, B vitamins, and probiotics, have been associated with improved mood and mental health. We will discuss gut-healthy foods and dietary strategies that can support emotional well-being and help individuals manage emotional eating tendencies.

- Seeking Support: Professional Help for Emotional Eating:

We will discuss the importance of seeking professional help when addressing emotional eating patterns that may be impacting gut health and overall well-being. Registered dietitians, therapists, and other healthcare professionals can provide guidance, support, and evidence-based interventions to help individuals develop healthier coping mechanisms and establish a positive relationship with food.

Recognizing the complex relationship between emotional eating, gut health, and emotional well-being is crucial for individuals seeking to address emotional eating patterns. By understanding the gut-brain axis, managing stress, cultivating mindful eating practices, and nourishing the gut with appropriate nutrition, individuals can develop healthier coping mechanisms and support a balanced gut microbiome. This, in turn, can contribute to improved emotional well-being and a reduced reliance on emotional eating behaviors.

8.5 Sustaining a Healthy Gut for Long-Term Weight Management

Maintaining a healthy gut is not only essential for overall well-being but also plays a significant role in long-term weight management. In this chapter, "Sustaining a Healthy Gut for Long-Term Weight Management," we will explore the connection between gut health and weight, focusing on strategies to support a healthy gut microbiome for sustainable weight management.

- Gut Health and Weight Regulation:

We will discuss the intricate relationship between gut health and weight regulation. The gut microbiome influences various aspects of metabolism, including energy extraction from food, fat storage, and appetite regulation. We will explore how an imbalanced gut microbiome can contribute to weight gain and the development of obesity.

- Gut Microbiome and Metabolic Health:

We will delve into the role of the gut microbiome in metabolic health. The composition and diversity of gut bacteria have been linked to insulin sensitivity, glucose metabolism, and lipid metabolism. We will discuss how an unhealthy gut microbiome can lead to metabolic dysregulation and weight-related health issues.

- Dietary Factors for a Healthy Gut and Weight Management:

We will explore dietary strategies that promote both a healthy gut and sustainable weight management. This includes emphasizing whole, unprocessed foods rich in fiber, prebiotics, and plant-based nutrients. We will also discuss the importance of reducing excessive sugar, refined carbohydrates, and artificial additives that can negatively impact the gut microbiome and contribute to weight gain.

- Physical Activity and Gut Health:

We will examine the role of physical activity in supporting a healthy gut and weight management. Regular exercise has been shown to positively influence the composition and diversity of gut bacteria, enhance gut barrier function, and improve metabolic health. We will discuss the types and duration of exercise that can benefit the gut microbiome and aid in weight management.

- Sleep and Gut Health:

We will discuss the importance of quality sleep for both gut health and weight management. Sleep deprivation and disturbances have been associated with alterations in the gut microbiome, increased appetite, and weight gain. We will explore strategies for optimizing sleep hygiene and establishing healthy sleep patterns to support a balanced gut and overall weight management.

- **Stress Management and Gut Health:**
We will explore the impact of stress on gut health and weight management. Chronic stress can disrupt the gut microbiome, promote inflammation, and contribute to weight gain. We will discuss stress management techniques such as mindfulness, meditation, and relaxation exercises that can help reduce stress levels and support a healthy gut for long-term weight management.
- **Sustainable Lifestyle Changes for Gut Health and Weight Management:**
We will discuss the importance of sustainable lifestyle changes in achieving and maintaining a healthy gut and weight. Crash diets and extreme approaches often fail to produce long-term results. We will explore the significance of gradual and sustainable changes in diet, physical activity, stress management, and sleep habits to promote a healthy gut and support weight management over time.
- **Gut Health Maintenance Strategies:**
We will provide practical strategies for maintaining a healthy gut microbiome in the long term. This includes regular consumption of fermented foods, incorporating prebiotic-rich foods into the diet, avoiding unnecessary antibiotic use, and adopting a diverse and plant-based eating pattern. We will also discuss the potential role of probiotic supplements in supporting gut health and weight management.

Sustaining a healthy gut is a key component of long-term weight management. By prioritizing dietary choices that nourish the gut microbiome, engaging in regular physical activity, managing stress levels, prioritizing quality sleep, and embracing sustainable lifestyle changes, individuals can establish a foundation for a healthy gut and sustainable weight management. The combination of a balanced gut microbiome and healthy lifestyle habits sets the stage for long-term success in maintaining a healthy weight and overall well-being.

Chapter 9

Gut Health and Immunity

9.1 The Gut's Role in Immune System Function

The gut plays a crucial role in the functioning of our immune system. In this chapter, "The Gut's Role in Immune System Function," we will explore the intricate connection between gut health and immunity. We will delve into the ways in which the gut microbiome and gut-associated lymphoid tissue (GALT) work together to support immune function and protect us from harmful pathogens.

- The Gut Microbiome and Immune System Crosstalk:

We will discuss how the gut microbiome interacts with the immune system, forming a complex network of communication and interaction. The gut microbiome helps train and modulate the immune system, playing a critical role in distinguishing between harmful pathogens and beneficial microorganisms. We will explore the impact of a balanced gut microbiome on immune cell development, activation, and response.

- Gut Permeability and Immune Activation:

We will explore the concept of gut permeability and its influence on immune system activation. When the gut barrier becomes compromised, toxins and pathogens can enter the bloodstream, triggering an immune response and potentially leading to chronic inflammation. We will discuss the factors that contribute to gut permeability and its implications for immune health.

- Gut-Associated Lymphoid Tissue (GALT):

We will delve into the gut-associated lymphoid tissue (GALT), a specialized part of the immune system located in the gut. GALT includes various structures such as Peyer's patches, mesenteric lymph nodes, and lymphoid follicles.

We will explore the functions of GALT in immune surveillance, antigen sampling, and immune response regulation.

- Gut Microbiome Diversity and Immune Resilience: We will discuss the importance of gut microbiome diversity in maintaining immune resilience. A diverse gut microbiome supports a balanced immune response, reduces the risk of allergies and autoimmune conditions, and enhances the body's ability to fight off infections. We will explore strategies for promoting gut microbiome diversity through diet, lifestyle, and probiotic interventions.
- Immune-Boosting Nutrients for Gut Health: We will explore specific nutrients that play a vital role in supporting gut health and immune function. This includes vitamins (such as vitamin C, D, and A), minerals (such as zinc and selenium), and other bioactive compounds found in various foods. We will discuss the sources of these nutrients and their impact on gut health and immune system resilience.
- Gut Health, Inflammation, and Autoimmune Conditions: We will examine the relationship between gut health, inflammation, and autoimmune conditions. Imbalances in the gut microbiome and increased gut permeability can contribute to chronic inflammation, which may trigger or exacerbate autoimmune disorders. We will discuss the potential of gut-targeted interventions in managing autoimmune conditions and reducing inflammation.
- Probiotics and Immune Health: We will explore the role of probiotics in promoting immune health and modulating immune responses. Probiotics, beneficial bacteria that can be consumed through food or supplements, have been shown to support gut health and enhance immune function. We will discuss the specific strains of probiotics that have demonstrated immune-modulating effects and their potential applications.
- Gut Health and Vaccinations:

We will discuss the influence of gut health on vaccine efficacy. A healthy gut microbiome and robust immune system are essential for optimal vaccine responses. We will explore the emerging field of research on the gut microbiome's impact on vaccine outcomes and discuss strategies to support gut health before and after vaccinations.

The gut and immune system are intricately interconnected, and maintaining a healthy gut is crucial for robust immune function. By understanding the role of the gut microbiome, gut-associated lymphoid tissue, and gut permeability in immune system function, individuals can adopt strategies to support their gut health and enhance immune resilience. Through a combination of dietary choices, lifestyle practices, and targeted interventions, we can optimize gut health and strengthen our immune system to protect against pathogens and promote overall well-being.

9.2 Gut Health and Autoimmune Conditions

In this chapter, "Gut Health and Autoimmune Conditions," we will explore the fascinating link between gut health and autoimmune conditions. Autoimmune diseases occur when the immune system mistakenly attacks healthy cells in the body, leading to chronic inflammation and tissue damage. Emerging research suggests that imbalances in the gut microbiome and increased gut permeability play a significant role in the development and progression of autoimmune conditions. By understanding the complex relationship between the gut and autoimmune diseases, we can explore strategies to promote gut health and potentially mitigate the risk and severity of autoimmune conditions.

- The Gut Microbiome and Autoimmunity: We will examine the impact of the gut microbiome on autoimmune diseases. The gut microbiome plays a critical role in immune system regulation and tolerance, helping to distinguish between harmful pathogens and beneficial microorganisms. We will explore the role of specific gut bacteria in autoimmune conditions and discuss the mechanisms by which the gut microbiome influences immune responses.

- Gut Permeability and Autoimmune Disorders: We will delve into the concept of gut permeability, commonly referred to as "leaky gut," and its association with autoimmune diseases. Increased intestinal permeability can allow harmful substances to enter the bloodstream, triggering immune responses and contributing to chronic inflammation. We will explore the potential mechanisms linking gut permeability with the development and progression of autoimmune conditions.
- Dysbiosis and Autoimmunity: We will discuss the concept of dysbiosis, an imbalance in the gut microbiome composition, and its implications for autoimmune diseases. Dysbiosis can disrupt immune system regulation and promote inflammation, potentially triggering or exacerbating autoimmune conditions. We will explore the factors that contribute to dysbiosis and discuss strategies to restore a healthy balance of gut bacteria.
- Molecular Mimicry and Autoimmunity: We will explore the concept of molecular mimicry, a phenomenon in which certain components of the gut microbiome resemble host tissues, leading to cross-reactivity by the immune system. Molecular mimicry can trigger autoimmune responses as the immune system mistakenly attacks both the harmful bacteria and the host tissues. We will discuss the potential role of molecular mimicry in autoimmune diseases and its implications for gut health.
- Gut Health Interventions for Autoimmune Conditions: We will explore various gut health interventions that may help manage autoimmune conditions. This includes dietary modifications, such as eliminating potential trigger foods and incorporating anti-inflammatory and gut-supportive nutrients. We will also discuss the potential benefits of

probiotics, prebiotics, and other gut-targeted therapies in modulating immune responses and reducing autoimmune symptoms.

- Gut Health and Autoimmune Disease Management:

We will discuss the role of gut health in the management of autoimmune conditions. While gut health interventions cannot cure autoimmune diseases, they may help reduce inflammation, alleviate symptoms, and potentially slow disease progression. We will explore the importance of personalized approaches in managing autoimmune conditions and the potential synergistic effects of combining traditional medical treatments with gut-targeted interventions.

- Gut Health and Autoimmune Prevention:

We will examine the potential for gut health strategies in preventing autoimmune conditions. By promoting a balanced gut microbiome, maintaining gut barrier integrity, and reducing inflammation, individuals may be able to mitigate the risk of developing autoimmune diseases. We will discuss the importance of early intervention, lifestyle factors, and potential future directions in autoimmune prevention research.

The link between gut health and autoimmune conditions offers new insights into the complexity of autoimmune diseases. By understanding the role of the gut microbiome, gut permeability, dysbiosis, and molecular mimicry, individuals can explore interventions to support gut health and potentially mitigate the risk and severity of autoimmune conditions. While further research is needed, optimizing gut health may offer a promising avenue for improving the lives of individuals affected by autoimmune diseases.

9.3 Gut Health and Allergies

In this chapter, "Gut Health and Allergies," we will explore
the intricate relationship between gut health and allergic
conditions. Allergies are immune responses triggered by
normally harmless substances, such as pollen, dust mites,
or certain foods. Emerging research suggests that the health
of our gut plays a significant role in the development and
management of allergies. By understanding the complex
interplay between the gut microbiome, immune system, and
allergic responses, we can explore strategies to promote gut
health and potentially alleviate allergy symptoms.
•   Gut Microbiome and Allergies:
We will examine the influence of the gut microbiome on
allergic conditions. The gut microbiome consists of trillions
of microorganisms that reside in our intestines, influencing
various aspects of our health, including our immune system.
We will discuss how alterations in the gut microbiome
composition, such as reduced microbial diversity or
imbalances in specific bacterial species, may contribute to
the development of allergies.
•   Gut Permeability and Allergic Sensitization:
We will explore the concept of gut permeability, often
referred to as "leaky gut," and its association with allergic
sensitization. Increased intestinal permeability can allow
allergenic substances to enter the bloodstream more easily,
triggering immune responses and potentially leading to the
development of allergies. We will discuss the mechanisms
by which gut permeability influences allergic sensitization
and the importance of maintaining a healthy gut barrier.
•   Gut Immune System and Allergic Responses:
We will delve into the role of the gut immune system in
regulating allergic responses. The gut contains a significant
portion of our immune system, including specialized
immune cells that interact with the gut microbiome and help
shape immune responses. We will explore how imbalances
in gut immune function can contribute to allergic conditions

and discuss strategies to modulate the gut immune system for better allergy management.

- Gut Health Interventions for Allergies: We will discuss various gut health interventions that may help alleviate allergy symptoms. This includes dietary modifications, such as identifying and avoiding allergenic foods, as well as incorporating gut-supportive nutrients and probiotics. We will also explore the potential benefits of prebiotics, which can selectively promote the growth of beneficial gut bacteria, and their role in allergy prevention and management.
- Gut-Brain Axis and Allergic Conditions: We will explore the connection between the gut and the brain, known as the gut-brain axis, and its impact on allergic conditions. Communication between the gut and the brain occurs through neural, hormonal, and immune pathways, and disruptions in this communication may influence the development and severity of allergies. We will discuss the potential role of stress, emotions, and psychological factors in allergic responses and explore mind-body interventions for allergy management.
- Early Life Gut Health and Allergy Prevention: We will examine the importance of gut health during early life in preventing allergies. Research suggests that the development of a healthy gut microbiome in infancy and early childhood can have long-term implications for allergy risk. We will discuss the factors that contribute to healthy gut development in early life, including breastfeeding, exposure to diverse microbial environments, and avoiding unnecessary antibiotic use.
- Gut Health and Allergy Management: We will discuss the role of gut health in the management of existing allergies. While gut health interventions cannot cure allergies, they may help reduce inflammation, modulate immune responses, and potentially alleviate allergy symptoms. We will explore the importance of personalized approaches in allergy management and the potential

synergy between traditional allergy treatments and gut-targeted interventions.

The intricate relationship between gut health and allergies highlights the potential for gut-focused strategies in allergy prevention and management. By promoting a healthy gut microbiome, maintaining gut barrier integrity, modulating the gut immune system, and considering the gut-brain axis, individuals with allergies may find new avenues for improving their quality of life. Through ongoing research and a comprehensive understanding of the gut-allergy connection, we can continue to develop innovative approaches to tackle allergic conditions from a gut-centric perspective.
Do you agree with the table of contents for Chapter 9?

9.4 Boosting Immunity through Gut Nourishment

In this chapter, "Boosting Immunity through Gut Nourishment," we will explore the critical role of gut nourishment in enhancing and supporting a robust immune system. The health of our gut has a direct impact on the functioning of our immune system, and by focusing on nourishing the gut, we can optimize our body's defenses against pathogens, infections, and diseases. By understanding the key nutrients, foods, and lifestyle factors that contribute to a healthy gut and immune system, we can adopt strategies to boost our immunity and promote overall well-being.
- The Gut-Immune System Connection:
We will explore the intricate connection between the gut and the immune system. The gut houses a significant portion of our immune cells and plays a vital role in immune function. We will discuss how the gut acts as a barrier against pathogens, the influence of the gut microbiota on immune responses, and the communication pathways between the gut and immune system.
- Essential Nutrients for Immune Support:

We will delve into the specific nutrients that are essential for optimal immune function. This includes vitamins (such as vitamin C, vitamin D, and vitamin E), minerals (such as zinc and selenium), and other bioactive compounds (such as antioxidants and polyphenols). We will discuss the food sources that provide these nutrients and their role in supporting immune health.

- Gut-Boosting Foods for Immunity:

We will explore a variety of foods that can nourish and support a healthy gut, consequently boosting immunity. This includes a focus on plant-based foods rich in fiber, prebiotics, and probiotics. We will discuss the benefits of incorporating fruits, vegetables, whole grains, legumes, fermented foods, and other gut-friendly options into our diet to promote immune resilience.

- The Impact of Gut Health on Systemic Inflammation:

We will examine how gut health influences systemic inflammation, a critical factor in immune response. Chronic inflammation can impair immune function and make us more susceptible to infections and diseases. We will explore the connection between gut dysbiosis, intestinal permeability, and low-grade inflammation, and discuss dietary and lifestyle strategies to reduce inflammation and promote gut health.

- Gut Health, Stress, and Immune Function:

We will discuss the impact of stress on gut health and immune function. Chronic stress can disrupt the balance of the gut microbiota, compromise gut integrity, and impair immune responses. We will explore stress reduction techniques, such as mindfulness, meditation, and stress management strategies, to support both gut health and immune function.

- Lifestyle Factors for Gut Nourishment and Immune Support:

We will examine various lifestyle factors that contribute to gut nourishment and immune support. This includes regular physical activity, adequate sleep, hydration, and avoiding harmful habits like smoking and excessive alcohol consumption. We will discuss the positive effects of these lifestyle factors on gut health and immunity and provide practical tips for incorporating them into daily life.

- Gut Health, Chronic Diseases, and Immune Function:

We will explore the relationship between gut health, chronic diseases, and immune function. Certain chronic conditions, such as obesity, diabetes, and cardiovascular disease, can impact gut health and immune responses. We will discuss the role of gut-focused interventions in managing these conditions, improving immune function, and reducing the risk of complications.

Nourishing our gut is an essential component of boosting our immune system and promoting overall health and well-being. By focusing on the nutrients, foods, and lifestyle factors that support gut health, we can enhance immune function, reduce the risk of infections and diseases, and achieve a state of optimal well-being. By embracing a gut-nourishing approach to immune support, we empower ourselves to take charge of our health and cultivate resilience from within.

Chapter 10

Sugar and Gut health

10.1 parasites in sugar and their effect on gut and mental well being

Parasites are organisms that live and feed off other organisms, and they can enter the body through various sources, including contaminated food and water. While it's uncommon for parasites to be directly present in sugar, certain parasites can thrive in the gut when an individual consumes contaminated food or beverages, which may include sugar as an ingredient.

When parasites infect the gut, they can cause a range of symptoms and health issues. These symptoms may include abdominal pain, diarrhea, bloating, nausea, and fatigue. In severe cases or prolonged infections, parasites can lead to nutrient deficiencies, weight loss, and weakened immune function.

Regarding mental well-being, some research suggests that gut health, including the presence of parasites, can have an indirect impact on mental health. The gut-brain axis, which is the bidirectional communication network between the gut and the brain, plays a crucial role in regulating emotions and mental well-being. Disruptions in the gut microbiota balance, including the presence of parasites, may contribute to gut inflammation and affect the gut-brain communication, potentially leading to changes in mood, cognition, and behavior.

However, it's important to note that the relationship between parasites, gut health, and mental well-being is still an active area of research, and more studies are needed to fully understand the mechanisms involved and the extent of their impact.

If you're interested in exploring this topic further, I recommend consulting reputable scientific literature, medical journals, and research studies that focus on parasitic infections, gut health, and mental well-being. These sources can provide you with more specific and detailed information, including any potential links between parasites in sugar and their effects on gut health and mental well-being.

Please keep in mind that if you suspect you have a parasitic infection or any health concerns, it is important to consult with a healthcare professional for an accurate diagnosis and appropriate treatment.

10.2 how is gut microbiome affected by sugar

The gut microbiome, which refers to the community of microorganisms that reside in our digestive tract, can be influenced by various factors, including diet. Sugar consumption is one factor that can affect the composition and diversity of the gut microbiome.

- Increased Growth of Harmful Bacteria: Sugar, particularly refined sugars like sucrose and high-fructose corn syrup, can serve as a food source for certain pathogenic or harmful bacteria in the gut. These bacteria, such as Clostridium difficile and some strains of Escherichia coli, thrive on sugar and can proliferate, potentially leading to an imbalance in the gut microbiome.

- Reduced Diversity: A diet high in sugar and low in fiber can contribute to a decrease in the overall diversity of the gut microbiome. Fiber-rich foods, such as fruits, vegetables, and whole grains, support the growth of beneficial bacteria that promote a healthy gut environment. When sugar consumption is high and fiber intake is low, the growth of beneficial bacteria may be compromised, leading to a less diverse gut microbiome.

- Imbalance in Gut Microbial Metabolism: Sugar consumption can also affect the metabolic activities of the gut microbiome. Certain bacteria have the ability to break down complex carbohydrates and fiber, producing short-chain fatty acids (SCFAs) like butyrate, acetate, and propionate, which have beneficial effects on gut health. However, when the diet is high in sugar and low in fiber, there may be a shift in the metabolic activity of the gut microbiome, leading to a decrease in SCFA production and potentially impacting gut health.

- Inflammation and Gut Barrier Function: Excessive sugar consumption has been associated with chronic low-grade inflammation, which can affect gut barrier function. The gut barrier acts as a protective barrier, preventing harmful substances from crossing into the bloodstream. Disruptions in gut barrier function can lead to increased intestinal permeability (leaky gut), allowing unwanted substances to enter the bloodstream and potentially triggering immune responses and inflammation.

It's important to note that the effects of sugar on the gut microbiome can vary among individuals, depending on factors such as overall diet, genetics, and gut microbial composition. Additionally, moderate sugar consumption as part of a balanced diet may not have significant negative effects on the gut microbiome. However, excessive consumption of added sugars, particularly in the form of processed foods and beverages, can have detrimental effects on gut health.

To maintain a healthy gut microbiome, it is generally recommended to consume a varied diet rich in fiber from fruits, vegetables, whole grains, and legumes, while limiting added sugars and processed foods. This helps support the growth of beneficial bacteria and promote a diverse and balanced gut microbiome.

For more in-depth information and specific research studies on the effects of sugar on the gut microbiome, I recommend referring to scientific literature and reputable sources in the fields of gastroenterology, microbiology, and nutrition.

10.3 how does sugar intake affect the immunity of a person

Sugar intake can have various effects on the immune system, and excessive consumption of added sugars has been associated with negative impacts on immune function. Here are some ways in which sugar intake can affect immunity:

- Suppression of Immune Cells: High sugar intake, especially in the form of added sugars, has been shown to suppress the activity of certain immune cells, such as neutrophils, which are important for fighting bacterial infections. Consuming large amounts of sugar can impair the ability of immune cells to effectively respond to pathogens, leading to a weakened immune response.
- Increased Inflammation: Excessive sugar consumption can contribute to chronic low-grade inflammation in the body. Inflammation is a natural immune response to protect against harmful stimuli, but when it becomes chronic, it can disrupt immune system functioning. Prolonged inflammation can weaken the immune system, making it more difficult to fight off infections and increasing the risk of chronic diseases.
- Imbalanced Gut Microbiome: Sugar consumption can impact the balance of gut bacteria and the gut microbiome, which plays a critical role in immune system development and function. Excessive sugar intake can promote the growth of harmful bacteria in the gut while reducing the abundance of beneficial bacteria. This imbalance in the gut microbiome can compromise immune function and increase susceptibility to infections.
- Impaired Antioxidant Defense: High sugar intake can lead to increased production of reactive oxygen species (ROS) in the body. ROS are natural byproducts of cellular metabolism but can be harmful when their production exceeds the body's antioxidant defense mechanisms. Excessive sugar consumption can overwhelm the antioxidant system, leading to oxidative

stress and damage to immune cells, impairing their function.

- Nutrient Imbalances: Foods high in added sugars often lack essential nutrients, such as vitamins, minerals, and antioxidants, that are important for supporting a healthy immune system. Consuming excessive amounts of sugary foods and beverages can displace nutrient-dense foods from the diet, leading to nutrient imbalances and compromising immune function.

It's important to note that the negative effects of sugar on immunity are typically associated with excessive consumption of added sugars and not with naturally occurring sugars found in whole foods like fruits and vegetables. Moderation and balance in sugar intake are key to maintaining a healthy immune system.

A well-rounded, nutrient-dense diet that includes a variety of fruits, vegetables, whole grains, lean proteins, and healthy fats is generally recommended to support optimal immune function. Minimizing the intake of processed foods, sugary snacks, and sweetened beverages can help maintain a balanced immune response and overall health.

For more detailed and specific information on the effects of sugar on immunity, I suggest referring to scientific literature and reputable sources in the fields of immunology, nutrition, and human physiology.

10.4 l glutamine and its effect on sugar cravings

L-glutamine is an amino acid that plays several roles in the body, including its involvement in the regulation of sugar cravings. Here are some key points regarding L-glutamine and its potential effects on sugar cravings

- Brain Fuel: L-glutamine is considered a conditionally essential amino acid, meaning that under certain circumstances, such as during times of stress or illness, the body may require more L-glutamine than it can produce. L-glutamine serves as a primary source of fuel for the brain, and maintaining adequate levels of L-glutamine may help support healthy brain function, including the regulation of cravings.

- Blood Sugar Regulation: L-glutamine has been suggested to support stable blood sugar levels. When blood sugar levels drop, it can trigger cravings for quick sources of energy, such as sugary foods. By helping to maintain stable blood sugar levels, L-glutamine may indirectly help reduce sugar cravings.

- Gut Health: L-glutamine is beneficial for maintaining the health and integrity of the gut lining. The gut lining acts as a barrier, preventing harmful substances from entering the bloodstream. When the gut lining is compromised, it can lead to increased inflammation and potential nutrient deficiencies, which may contribute to sugar cravings. By supporting gut health, L-glutamine may help reduce cravings for sugar and other unhealthy foods.

- Dopamine Regulation: L-glutamine is involved in the synthesis of neurotransmitters, including dopamine. Dopamine plays a role in reward pathways and pleasure sensations in the brain. Imbalances in dopamine signaling have been linked to cravings and addictive behaviors, including sugar cravings. While the exact mechanisms are not fully understood, L-glutamine may help maintain balanced dopamine levels, potentially reducing sugar cravings.

- Individual Variations: It's important to note that individual responses to L-glutamine may vary. While some people may find L-glutamine supplementation helpful in reducing sugar cravings, others may not experience the same effects. Factors such as overall diet, lifestyle, and underlying health conditions can influence the effectiveness of L-glutamine in managing sugar cravings.

It's always recommended to consult with a healthcare professional before starting any new supplement regimen. They can provide personalized advice based on your

specific health needs and guide you on the appropriate dosage and duration of L-glutamine supplementation.
For more comprehensive information on L-glutamine and its effects on sugar cravings, I suggest referring to scientific literature and consulting reputable sources in the fields of nutrition, biochemistry, and neuroscience.

Chapter 11

<u>Gluten and its effect on gut health</u>

11.1 Effects of gluten on gut health

Gluten is a protein found in certain grains, such as wheat, barley, and rye. For individuals with celiac disease or non-celiac gluten sensitivity, consuming gluten can have significant effects on gut health. Here are some key points regarding gluten and its impact on the gut:

- Celiac Disease: Celiac disease is an autoimmune disorder triggered by the ingestion of gluten. In individuals with celiac disease, the immune system responds abnormally to gluten, leading to inflammation and damage to the lining of the small intestine. This can result in various gastrointestinal symptoms, including diarrhea, abdominal pain, bloating, and malabsorption of nutrients. Long-term untreated celiac disease can lead to nutrient deficiencies, weight loss, and other complications.

- Non-Celiac Gluten Sensitivity: Some individuals may experience symptoms similar to celiac disease, such as gastrointestinal issues and fatigue, after consuming gluten-containing foods, even without having celiac disease. This condition is known as non-celiac gluten sensitivity. While the exact mechanisms are not fully understood, it is believed that non-celiac gluten sensitivity involves an immune response or other sensitivity reactions to gluten. The symptoms can vary and may also include brain fog, joint pain, and skin problems.

- Gut Inflammation and Intestinal Permeability: Gluten can trigger inflammation in the gut, particularly in individuals with celiac disease or gluten sensitivity. This inflammation can disrupt the integrity of the intestinal lining, leading to increased intestinal permeability, often referred to as "leaky gut." When the intestinal barrier becomes compromised, it allows larger molecules, toxins, and bacteria to pass through into the bloodstream, potentially triggering immune responses and inflammation in other parts of the body.

- Altered Gut Microbiome: Gluten consumption may also impact the composition of the gut microbiome, the community of microorganisms living in the digestive tract. Studies have shown that individuals with celiac disease or non-celiac gluten sensitivity may have differences in their gut microbial profiles compared to those without these conditions. Imbalances in the gut microbiome have been associated with various digestive issues and immune dysregulation.

- Other Factors: It's important to note that not everyone experiences negative effects from gluten consumption. The majority of people can tolerate gluten without any adverse reactions. For those without celiac disease or non-celiac gluten sensitivity, avoiding gluten is generally unnecessary and may even lead to a restrictive diet that lacks certain nutrients found in gluten-containing grains.

If you suspect that you have celiac disease or gluten sensitivity, it is recommended to consult with a healthcare professional for proper evaluation and diagnosis. They can guide you through the necessary testing and help you develop an appropriate dietary plan.

For more in-depth information and specific research studies on gluten and its effects on gut health, I suggest referring to scientific literature and reputable sources in the fields of gastroenterology, immunology, and nutrition.

11.2 gut health and depression

There is growing evidence to suggest a link between gut health and depression, highlighting the importance of a healthy gut microbiome for mental well-being. Here are some key points regarding the relationship between gut health and depression:

- Gut-Brain Axis: The gut and the brain are connected through a bidirectional communication pathway known as the gut-brain axis. The gut microbiome, which consists of trillions of microorganisms residing in the digestive tract, plays a crucial role in this communication. The gut microbiome produces various compounds and neurotransmitters that can influence brain function and mood.

- Serotonin Production: Serotonin is a neurotransmitter that is often referred to as the "feel-good" neurotransmitter. It plays a key role in regulating mood, appetite, and sleep. Interestingly, about 90% of serotonin is produced in the gut, primarily by certain bacteria in the gut microbiome. Imbalances in the gut microbiome can potentially impact serotonin production, which may contribute to mood disorders such as depression.

- Inflammation and Immune System Activation: The gut microbiome helps regulate the immune system and plays a role in maintaining a balanced inflammatory response. Chronic inflammation and immune system dysregulation have been associated with various mental health conditions, including depression. Imbalances in the gut microbiome can lead to increased intestinal permeability ("leaky gut"), allowing toxins and inflammatory molecules to enter the bloodstream and potentially affect brain function.

- Neurotransmitter Regulation: The gut microbiome can influence the production and metabolism of neurotransmitters other than serotonin, such as dopamine and gamma-aminobutyric acid (GABA), which are also involved in mood regulation. Imbalances in the gut microbiome may disrupt the production and balance of these neurotransmitters, potentially contributing to depressive symptoms.

- Stress Response: The gut microbiome can influence the body's response to stress. Chronic stress can negatively impact the gut microbiome, leading to dysbiosis (imbalanced microbial composition) and impaired gut barrier function. These changes can further contribute to inflammation and may influence the development or exacerbation of depressive symptoms.

While the relationship between gut health and depression is an active area of research, it's important to note that depression is a complex condition with multiple contributing factors. Addressing gut health alone may not be sufficient to treat depression, and a comprehensive approach that includes various strategies, such as therapy, medication (if necessary), and lifestyle modifications, is often recommended.

If you are experiencing symptoms of depression or have concerns about your mental health, it's essential to consult with a healthcare professional. They can provide a thorough evaluation, diagnose any underlying conditions, and recommend appropriate treatment options tailored to your specific needs.

For further information on the connection between gut health and depression, I recommend referring to scientific literature and reputable sources in the fields of psychiatry, neuroscience, and gastroenterology.

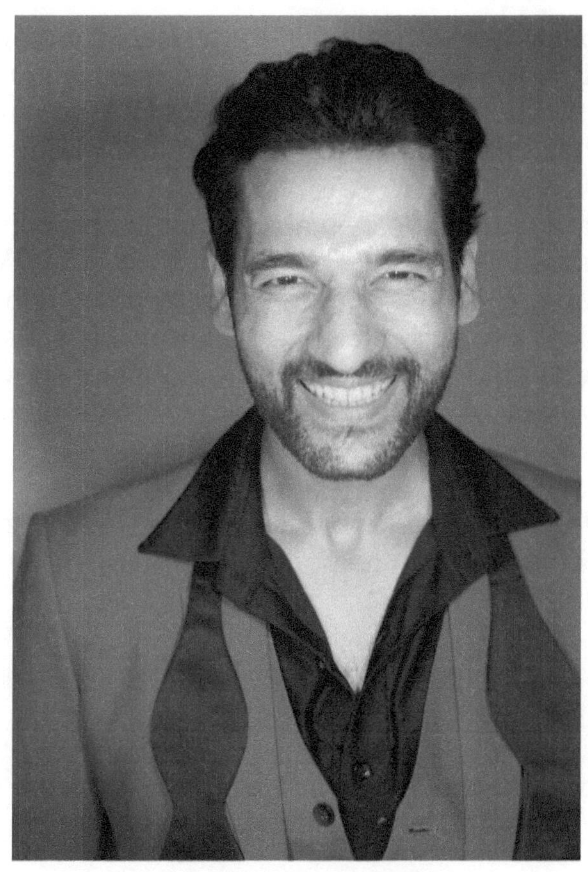

About the Author

Umesh Pherwani is a life coach a NLP trainer and a keynote speaker.

His first book 'Are you out of your mind' was very well received and marked his first steps into the literary world.

Born in Mumbai, he completed his Masters in Psychology and is pursuing a Ph.D. in the same line of study. Umesh completed a 125 hours program in neuroscience and the neurobiology of behavior from Stanford university.

He previously worked as a flight attendant for eleven years with KLM- Northwest Airlines. This coupled with his current profession, where he conducts regular NLP seminars globally, has enabled him to travel extensively.

The multi-faceted Umesh is also a model and actor—his most famous show being Family No. 1 on Sony TV. Roll Sound Camera Action, a feature film awaiting release, will see him play the lead. A born entertainer, he is also a stand-up comedian and has performed to houseful shows in Mumbai, Dubai, Abu Dhabi, Bangkok, Amsterdam and St. Martin.

Awards he's won include being bestowed with the title Mr. Popular, which he won as part of the Grasim Mr. India pageant in 2003.

During his spare time, Umesh loves to write and has a food and lifestyle blog.

Umesh loves to take on new challenges, he went on to lose 32 kgs in 3 months after following a strict diet and workout regime.
His second book was The Mind Switch which was the first in the trio series, followed by The Body Switch and The Gut Switch.

Umesh has also authored a fiction novel 'Shadows Embrace' which is a fast faced spy thriller. It is an electrifying tale that explores the complex dynamic of love,duty and sacrifice in the world of espionage.